AUTIST

PSYCHEDELIC

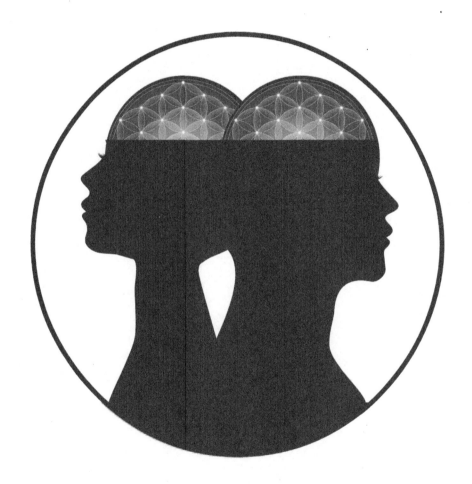

THE SELF-REPORTED BENEFITS & CHALLENGES OF EXPERIENCING LSD, MDMA, PSILOCYBIN, & OTHER PSYCHEDELICS AS TOLD BY NEURODIVERGENT ADULTS NAVIGATING ADHD, ALEXITHYMIA, ANXIETY, ASPERGER'S, AUTISM, DEPRESSION, OCD, PTSD & OTHER CONDITIONS

EDITOR'S NOTE

This book relates the events surrounding the use of various psychoactive chemical compounds and substances including 2,5-dimethoxy-4-bromophenethylamine (2C-B), ketamine, 3,4,5-trimethoxyphenethylamine (Mescaline, as within Peyote, San Pedro cacti), N,N-dimethyltryptamine (DMT), lysergic acid diethylamide (LSD), 3,4-methylenedioxyamphetamine (MDA), 3,4-Methylenedioxymethamphetamine (MDMA), psilocybin (as within psychoactive mushrooms), tetrahydrocannabinol (THC), and 5-MeO-DMT. It is a federal criminal offense in the United States and many other countries, punishable by imprisonment and/or fines; to manufacture, cultivate, possess, share, and/or supply most of the aforementioned compounds and substances. Any reader should therefore understand that this book is presented for entertainment purposes only and is therefore not intended to encourage any reader to break the law. The editor and the publisher expressly disclaim any liability, loss, or risk, personal or otherwise, that is incurred as a consequence, directly or indirectly, of the use or application of any contents of this book.

Regarding edits made in this book: all message excerpts, essays and survey responses have been edited for the purposes of correcting spelling, cleaning up language translations, updating vague pronouns, and rearranging text for print layout purposes. Contributions were also edited to remove specific dose amounts (so as to not invite mimicry) and to also remove any identifying information — including but not limited to names, dates, locations, and any other information that could be used to implicate any contributors in the participation of illegal activities.

Regarding inclusions & exclusions: a total of 14 essays were received with all 14 included in final publish. A total of 36 survey responses were received with 27 included in final publish; 8 survey respondents were lost to followup; 1 survey response was also excluded as it did not involve the use of psychedelic substances.

Regarding views expressed in this book: any view or opinion expressed by any particular contributor — including the views and opinions expressed within the "Introduction", "Story So Far", "Autistic Psychedelic Scrapbook", "What Do You Want To Tell The World About Psychedelics & Autism?", "AutiticPsychedelic.com Qualitative Survey Responses", and "The Conversation Continues" portions of this book — is to be considered the sole expression of the specific contributor and does not necessarily reflect the views and opinions held by any of the other contributors nor any of the other members or organizers of the Autistic Psychedelic Community.

DEDICATION

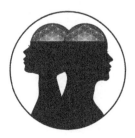

This book is dedicated to all those who've shared their stories, insights, time, and energy with everyone involved in the Autistic Psychedelic Community project; to all those autistics and neurodivergent individuals who felt compelled to share their perspectives in hopes that such perspectives could potentially serve to support the health and wellness of others.

Although the identities of these contributors have been made anonymous — for now, anyway — I proudly and graciously invite anyone reading this to join me in thanking these individuals for sharing such deeply personal truths. In doing so, these contributors have granted us the opportunity to expand our understandings of not only the potential benefits and challenges of psychedelic medicines, but also the nuanced complexities inherent in any particular neurodivergent perspective.

Every single one of these contributors is a hero — to me, anyway — and so also is anyone who may be willing to speak openly and honestly about these (hopefully formerly) stigmatized topics in the future. Because the more often we discuss such topics — together, in public — the more quickly we'll all be able to push beyond the present stigmas and enter into an era in which both neurodivergence and psychedelics can be more commonly understood, and in turn, navigated more intelligently.

With Love & Gratitude,
-Aaron Paul Orsini
Co-Founder, Co-Organizer & Co-Facilitator
Autistic Psychedelic Community

WORDS OF GRATITUDE FROM APC CO-FOUNDER JUSTINE LEE

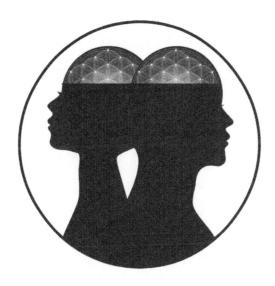

Some months ago, I left Aaron a comment in a Google Doc copy of a book he wrote and posted online. He'd requested help. I wasn't really sure what I had to offer but I reached out anyway.

The rest is history — unprecedented history, in fact. Yet it also seems like it's only just begun. There's still more history to be made — as well as more histories that ought to be told.

I've been happily offering my help to the Autistic Psychedelic Community alongside Aaron for more than a year now, grateful to have been able to give what I could.

Thank you to all those who have shared a bit of their histories. And thank you also to all those who are listening.

Love,

Justine :)
Co-Founder, Co-Organizer & Co-Facilitator
Autistic Psychedelic Community

TABLE OF CONTENTS

> *Chronological re-telling of the writing, publishing & first public keynote presentation of "Autism On Acid" as told through personal reflections & key emails excerpts that inspired the creation & founding of the Autistic Psychedelic Community in March of 2020....*

> *Additional email excerpts sourced from neurodivergent contributors featured alongside online Autistic Psychedelic Community video content made accessible via text-based links & scannable QR codes....*

> *14 personal essays & reflections written by neurodivergent contributors.*

> *27 neurodivergent contributors respond to a nine-question survey inquiring about how they perceived their lives & neurodivergence before, during & after their intentional use of various psychedelics.....*

INTRODUCTION

By Aaron Paul Orsini

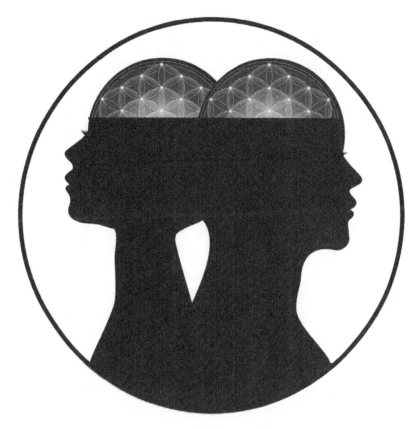

This book is a mixed-medium anthology featuring personal reflections, direct messages, emails, comments, essays, and survey responses collected from more than 40 neurodivergent individuals. There are many perspectives expressed within this text, and as you'll see as we progress through this work, the experiences described tend to be just as varied and diverse as the neurotypes and personalities and backgrounds and ages of the contributors themselves.

This book is also an open offering; a wide-reaching archive of the insights obtained as a result of the publishing of *Autism On Acid: How LSD Helped Me Understand, Navigate, Alter & Appreciate My Autistic Perceptions* in September, 2019, and the founding of the Autistic Psychedelic Community in March, 2020.

I'm writing this introduction in the early months of the year 2021. In the United States, Oregon voters just voted to legalize psilocybin-assisted therapy statewide, thus beginning a two-year rollout period in which the state will formulate a framework that could very well become a template for other states to follow. Also in the United States: MDMA-assisted therapy is nearly through the 3rd and final phase of its own clinical trials, and could soon become a legal, FDA-approved medicine in the United States. As the aforementioned legislative changes continue to develop, it's also worth remembering that there are already countless centers presently offering psychedelic sessions in monitored, medically screened, and fully legal contexts made possible through religious and indigenous protections. In certain other countries such as Jamaica and the Netherlands, pre-standing laws continue to permit the opening and operation of increasingly robust psilocybin-based retreat centers and research facilities. And on stock markets all throughout the world, an explosion of new psychedelic-focused medicine companies are going public with an open declaration of the intent to study substances such as psilocybin and LSD and other novel compounds for specific medicinal and therapeutic purposes.

Put simply: the so-called "Psychedelic Renaissance" is now in full swing, and it doesn't appear to be slowing down anytime soon. And so if we are to continue down this path, it seems appropriate that stories, such as the ones contained in this book, be made more broadly available. Because by speaking our truths in public, we grant researchers and clinicians and healers from a variety of disciplines the chance to better understand the potential paths forward. In this way, this book is perhaps best framed as an offering to those who are presently researching the potential therapeutic and medicinal qualities of these substances.

Speaking of research.... let me also be clear in stating that this book is by no means intended to be a substitute for rigorous, peer-reviewed science. Relatedly: if you weren't already aware, I myself am not a credentialed scientist. Apart from holding a sustained special focus toward the intersection of psychedelics and neurodivergence over the last seven years, I hold no certifications nor relevant academic degrees as of this publishing.

Although I possess no official credentials in the psychedelic sciences, I remain nonetheless confident in discussing my own personal experiences, just as I remain confident as I stand behind all those who entrusted me with bringing their personal truths into public through the publishing of this anthology.

It's not everyday that individuals collectively agree to express personal truths in this manner, most especially truths that are most likely foreign to just about everyone who happens upon this book. This may seem like a fringe subject, but I assure you that the hundreds of messages in my inboxes prove otherwise.

The relative scarcity of publicly discussed neurodivergent psychedelic experiences makes sense when one considers the cultural container in which these experiences have been taking place. As of the release date of this book, it will have been exactly 50 years to the day since the prohibition of psilocybin and LSD went into effect in the United States on Saturday, May 1st, 1971. Throughout that same 50-year period, the neurodivergent conditions explored in this book have been gradually undergoing their own subtle shifts, moving from the stigmatized shadows of shame and pathology and otherness into the spotlight of cultural conversation, support, acceptance, and compassion. Even so, there is still more work to be done in the domains of both psychedelic and neurodivergent advocacy. There will always be more work to be done. Yes. And that work begins and expands whenever we do exactly what we're doing now: listening to all those who've lived these experiences, honoring their words, and giving thanks for their insights. Because by listening to these contributors, we set ourselves on a path toward more fully understanding what's possible in this emerging field of study.

As we advance through each perspective shared in this book, my hope is that researchers and mental health professionals and casual readers alike will be better able to gain insight into the complexity of neurodivergent psychedelic experiences, and general psychedelic experiences more broadly.

I similarly hope that by the time you have finished this book you will understand that not all psychedelic experiences result in nirvana.

These experiences are not always filled with pure love and light. And they're not always safe for everyone.

When utilized in a responsible and well-informed manner, psychedelics offer profound potential for insight, healing, and growth. When used in an irresponsible or uninformed manner, however, psychedelics present the very real potential of engendering psychological or physiological harm.

Now. Because I'm not a medical professional, I will abstain from speaking to the particulars and once again strongly advise — nay, absolutely 100% insist, from a place of loving care — that anyone considering psychedelic services seek out as complete of an understanding as possible regarding contraindications and other critical considerations before ever engaging with these tools. I don't say this to scare anyone. I say this because I care about you — all of you — deeply.

We've done so much as a species to bring ourselves closer and closer to the point of being able to safely and responsibly wield the psychedelic flame in more intelligent and calculated ways. And as we continue to advance through this so-called "Psychedelic Renaissance" — and complete the transition from a predominantly psychedelic-naive culture toward a more psychedelic-aware culture — my hope is that we can remain honest and open about all of the potential benefits *and* risks *and* challenges associated with these powerful molecules. Anything less than this level of open and honest conversation would be a deep disservice to all those who've worked so hard to understand and advocate and educate one another about these substances.

There's so much more I'd like to express about all of this, but I'll save that for another day. For now I'd like to close out with a brief piece of prose that I feel more fully expresses everything I've attempted to articulate through this introduction...

Psychedelic molecules are like fire. The fire can heal. The fire can harm. The fire can warm. The fire can be worshipped. The fire can be feared. The fire can be amazing to admire... for a while. The fire can humble, help, or hinder us. The fire can seem mysterious or magical or terrifying or unnecessary (at times) or critical (at other times). The fire can clear the forest to make way for new growth. The fire can glow brilliantly to illuminate the darkness. The fire can glow so bright that it blinds the eyes to dangers hidden in plain sight. Indeed. But regardless of which labels or descriptors or namings we assign to the psychedelic fire — "It's a *medicine*! It's a *drug*! It's a *sacrament*! It's a *miracle*! It's a *plant*! It's a *molecule*! It's a *chemical*! It's a *ineffable*!" — it seems wise to give ourselves the chance to fully study the fire; to respect it; to honor it; and understand it as best as we can. Because if we do that — and do that sincerely, with as much patience and diligence and compassion as possible — then we'll likewise give ourselves the chance to be able to wield the psychedelic flame with the same ease, confidence, and precautionary common sense that we've come to expect whenever any modern human wields any now-common candle, or matchstick, or campfire, or stovetop flame.

CONTENT WARNINGS

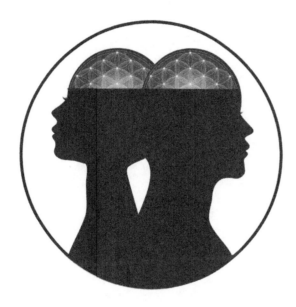

In the interest of supporting the reader's comfort and overall well-being — while still making a conscious and intentional editorial decision to lend a voice to those who contributed to this book regardless of their disclosure of choices made that could potentially result in adverse responses to psychedelic use — content warnings have been added throughout this book. These content warnings appear prior to the discussion of any especially challenging topics and/or the discussion of conditions, symptoms, dosages, or dose amounts associated with potential adverse responses to psychedelics. As an overall content warning, please note that the following potentially challenging topics will be discussed one or more times throughout the remainder of this book:

- Abuse
- Applied Behavior Analysis (ABA) Institutionalization
- Descriptions of Violence
- Hallucinogen Persisting Perception Disorder (HPPD)
- Near-Death Experiences (NDE)
- Self-Harm
- Suicide / Suicidal Ideation

FROM AUTISM ON ACID TO AUTISTIC PSYCHEDELIC

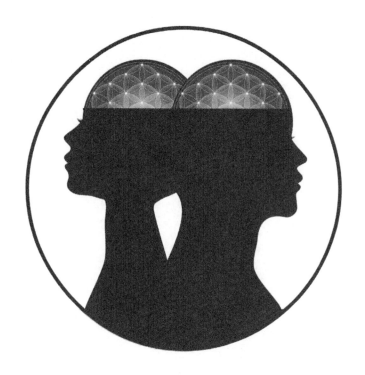

REFLECTIONS & EXCERPTS

FROM COMMUNITY CORRESPONDENCE

THE STORY SO FAR

By Aaron Paul Orsini

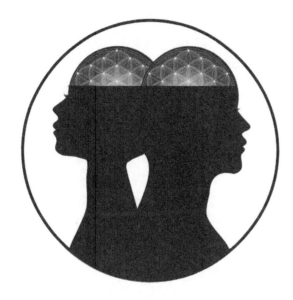

On the afternoon of September 17th, 2019, I sat in a thinly-padded square chair, in a big open reading room, at a Los Angeles public library, for 7 hours, rereading the same speech, over and over and over, while my partner sat opposite me, flipping through magazines, possibly bored but just as supportive as she had always been.

My partner and I had traveled down to Los Angeles by bus, staying at a nearby hotel that we had since checked out of that morning, meaning that at this particular point in time, we were carrying all of our luggages with us. So there we were — in the middle of the Los Angeles public library, surrounded by suitcases and backpacks — as my mind began racing, excited and anxious and uncertain about the upcoming consequences for my fastly approaching leap into public-facing advocacy.

I'd been invited by email to speak publicly that night about my book, *Autism on Acid*, as part of a presentation for the Southern California psychedelic society, the Aware Project (AwareProject.org), a group whose aim is "to balance the public conversation about psychedelics, spread accurate information, and give a new face to psychedelia."

I felt incredibly lucky to have been invited to share my story, especially as I stopped to recall all the times I'd felt so very close to fully abandoning the project in the previous years.

Fifteen months prior to that anxious afternoon in the L.A. library — in the summer of 2018, during one of my other unexpectedly pivotal visits to L.A. — I nervously attended my first psychedelic conference: the Los Angeles Psychedelic Science Symposium.

When I went to the conference, I had brought with me a box full of stapled-together copies of the still very rough and much more brief version of my full, eventually published book, *Autism On Acid*.

I had brought these DIY copies of my book — which I'd printed out at a local office supply store, much to the confusion of the employee assisting me at the printing center kiosk — with the intention of handing out copies to other conferencegoers. The funny thing was, though... I didn't have a table. I wasn't an invited speaker. I just figured, hey, these people are into this stuff. Maybe they'll be into my story (?).

After checking in at the registration desk on the morning of the conference, I felt full of anxious excitement, clutching my cardboard box full of books as I contemplated the weight of what I was there to do.

As the morning session unfolded, I sat in the back of the room. I watched a few speakers. I watched a few more. I thought to myself over and over "This is ridiculous. I should go home. No one wants to read a book about some autistic doing drugs. Yep. Okay. I should just go home."

And so when the lunch hour came, I left. I walked out of the conference hall, and I just, walked. Aimlessly. Anxiously. I walked.

My bus back home wasn't until very much later in that day, but in the moment — amidst that lunchtime walk — I was just, done. It was a really great idea, this whole bringing books to this conference thing. But no thanks. I didn't want that sort of attention. I didn't want to deal with the reactions of the people I would meet. So I walked away. And I was legitimately ready to just go and sit at the bus stop until my late-evening ride was set to arrive when I said to myself "Well, I came all the way here. I guess I'll just go and leave a few copies on some chairs or something."

So I walked back into the conference and I did something that went against every fiber of my culturally ashamed being: I began handing out copies of this deeply personal book to everyone I encountered — scientists, presenters, strangers, whoever. I even handed books to a few famous psychedelic figures whose work I'd followed for many years.

I scribbled a quick note on the back of each book and handed a copy to all of these heroes I had seen on Twitter and YouTube and Netflix; professionals whose work I had appreciated and grown through in such meaningful ways. It was great to meet them. Sure. But I was still struggling to find my words.

The funny thing was... at this point in my life, even though I'd worked out a great deal of my general social anxiety, this whole meeting the public thing still felt incredibly difficult. It was 2018, and even though I'd benefitted from psychedelics and grown a great deal in my own understanding of my life, my behaviors, and my relationship with my autism diagnosis, I was still holding on to a lot of yet-to-be-unpacked shame about both my diagnosis *and* my use of psychedelics. Even at a conference dedicated to psychedelics, I felt... odd. And so when I brought these topics up with strangers, even famous strangers who had made a career out of talking about psychedelics, I still felt very stressed and very anxious. Because it's not an everyday thing to say "Hi I'm autistic. I do illegal drugs. Nice to meet you!" But in this instance, that was basically what I was doing. It was nerve-wracking, to say the least.

"Hi, I wrote this. Here you go!"

"Hi, I've read every book you've written. I'm a big fan. Thank you. I also wrote a book. Here it is. Okay. Bye!"

"Hi. Book? Great. Bye!"

On and on. I did this throughout the afternoon, hoping that one of the books I'd handed out would result in something. Exactly what? I wasn't sure. I just needed to talk about it with someone, anyone.

At that point in my journey, I felt so overloaded with this sense of knowing something that seemed simultaneously so very important but also somehow entirely ridiculous — maybe even dangerous or I don't know, insane maybe?

Anyhow. There I was, walking around the conference room, clutching this cardboard box full of stapled-together books as though it was a box full of rare and delicate treasure.

I needed to birth my truth into the world. And I needed to convey both my story *and* my questions to those who could help me make sense of all of it. So I continued this nerve-wracking dance of outing myself as an autistic (who'd used Schedule I drugs), all throughout the afternoon.

"Hi, I wrote this. Here you go!"

"Hi nice to meet you. Yeah I know. Crazy right? Autistics on LSD. Yep. Wild. But hey — gotta go!"

On and on this went until I was out of time. The day ended. The conference closed up. I walked outside. And I took the bus back home.

And then, nothing.

No one wrote me any emails. No one visited the link to the Google Doc copy of the book that I'd linked to on the last page. Nothing.

For MORE THAN A YEAR, nothing.

From the summer of 2018 until the summer of 2019, I received exactly zero emails from anyone I'd spoken with at the conference. And that seemed to be proof enough that this whole idea was ridiculous.

So I didn't do much more about it after the conference. Throughout the remainder of 2018 and a good portion of 2019, I sorta just... let it all fade into the background, partly because my efforts seemed like a failure, but also because I still really dreaded the concept of going around telling people "Hey! I'm autistic! I do drugs!" So I sort of just set the whole project aside and spent some time enjoying the joyous life I felt so fortunate to have been able to live after decades of depression and anxiety.

At that exact point in time — as in, the summer of 2019 — my life entailed mainly just, working. I was the on-site general manager of a backpacker hostel, where I was tasked with greeting and hosting guests from all around the world, helping them to connect through social events and excursions and big meals shared in the communal dining room. It was a joy. Truly. And it was during this same time at the backpacker hostel that I also began to realize that more than needing any particular substance, what I needed most was community, connection, and purpose.

And that's such a major realization that I could probably write an entire book about that realization alone.

But I'll take pause on waxing nostalgic and get on with the point.

The reason why I've brought you on this journey from the summer of 2018 (when I went to the Los Angeles Psychedelic Science Symposium) to the summer of 2019 (when I was working at the backpacker hostel, feeling more or less fine with the whole book thing being forgotten) is to illustrate the tremendous weight of a single email I received from an incredibly caring human named Ashley.

Email from Ashley — July 27, 2019, 3:21pm

Aaron,

I was turned on to your book by a participant in one of the MAPS clinical trials. I run a psychedelic society in Southern California. I wanted to email you to share my appreciation for your bravery to do your own self research and to share your story. I hope that it inspires more research. Have you encountered other people that have had similar experiences? […]

Lastly, if you are ever in Los Angeles, Santa Barbara, or San Diego and would like to share your story to our community, let me know.

Warmly,
Ashley

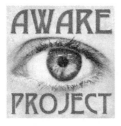

Ashley
Founder, Aware Project: Rethinking Psychedelics
www.awareproject.org

"No problem can be solved from the same level of consciousness that created it."
- Albert Einstein

Email Response to Ashley

July 27, 2019, 3:39pm

Wow. Hey Ashley! This is maybe the first email like this I've ever received so this really means a lot. I've been mostly underground w this story. I pushed it onto Amazon marketplace but then took it back down fearing repercussion. But emails like this matter a lot. You have no idea.

I've come across research correlating empathy increases and facial expression processing increases in subjects exposed to 5-HT2A Agonists (a term I'm trying to champion nowadays as a means of transcending stigmas and rooting this message in neuroscience).... and one of the most recently published theories from Robin Carhart-Harris likewise supported numerous theories... but as is the case with a lot of things psychedelic, truly rigorous research in this specific domain is yet to occur or receive funding [...]

In short, yes I would be thrilled to share my story or put together a more formal presentation. 5-HT2A Agonists have helped me to not only understand and overcome barriers inherent to autism but have also helped me access and process innumerable issues rooted in my otherwise inaccessible or trauma-walled-off memory bank. I can and have talked for hours about these subjects in small groups, and would be honored to present or participate in a panel, etc.

[I've] read probably no less than 300 academic texts in addition to the constant stream of published research and phenomenological reports that I consume regularly for the purpose of further refining my own theories.

I'll pause here because I could easily go on for very long, but in short… Yes. I live in San Diego and can easily commute to LA area if need be […] and a "coming out" such as this would really help me feel less alone in what I'm exploring.

With All The Gratitude Imaginable,
-Aaron

Ps I typed this excitedly on my phone so please excuse any typos :)

And that was it. That was the start. That was the spark that lit the fire of a passion project that is now poised to remain my central focus and mission for perhaps the rest of my life. And the main point I'm trying to make here is that all of this began with one email. I wrote the book, printed the copies, stapled them together, hauled them to a conference, got spooked, walked out without passing out a single copy, then walked back in to throw books at people in a hurried dance of embarrassment before leaving, going home, and not hearing anything from anyone for more than a year thereafter.

But then...THIS EMAIL.

Somehow or another, someone I had met at that conference had somehow eventually passed one of my stapled-together books to Ashley, which then lead to Ashley emailing me, which then lead to me saying "Yeah sure I'll speak at your group," which then lead to me sitting in the thinly padded chair at the LA public library on the morning of my presentation.

And so yes. There I was, sitting in the LA public library. And as I sat, I rehearsed the reading of no less than maybe 50 full pages of text — as in, 50 full 8.5" x 11" pages filled with double-spaced 10-point font that I thought I'd be able to read during that night's 75-minute presentation.

Spoiler alert: I did not get to all 50 pages.

To some people, 75 minutes might sound like a lot of time to fill. But given the amount of info I had amassed on the topic, and my autistic tendency to reeeeeally go deep on learning about my special interest subjects, 75 minutes seemed like barely more than enough time for my first outbreath. So I sat there, in the library, wondering about what might be the most important topic to cover...

Finally, after looping through the 50 or so odd pages over and over for hours and hours and hours, it was time to go.

I knew going into that night that the Aware Project would be recording the talk. I knew that the talk would likewise be broadcast live on Facebook. I knew that the edited recording would likewise be archived permanently on YouTube. And I also knew that I had just changed the status of my book from "Draft" to "Live", which meant that there was no means of turning back after that night's presentation.

From that day forward, everyone and anyone who Googled my name — including friends and family and potential employers, on and on — would see the words "Autism" and "LSD" on the very first page.

At the time, I didn't really know what to think about any of it. But that was also why I did it, too. I needed help. I needed support. I yearned for new and better answers. And I yearned for new and better questions.

So that night, I stood up in front of a room full of total strangers, and I said "Hi, My name is Aaron. At the age of 23, I was diagnosed with Autism Spectrum Disorder. At the age of 27, I was given Lysergic Acid Diethylamide..."

And what happened after that is as much a blur as it is a blessing.

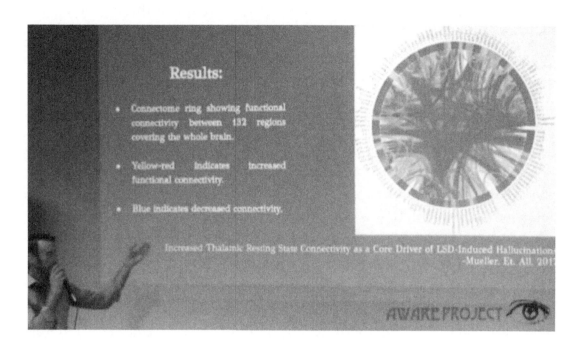

If you'd like, you can watch this presentation at this time.

Perhaps doing so will help you contextualize where we are in the story.

To view the presentation, please visit AutisticPsychedelic.com/video

— or —

Scan the QR Code on this page.

During the presentation, I did my best to speed through as much content as I could manage to cover. I presented some slides. I answered some questions. And then — after what felt like barely enough time to even begin to do justice to the weight of what I was there to discuss — my talk came to a close. I handed the microphone back to the host. I stepped aside. And then, something amazing happened...

A line formed.

It was a line of people. Only maybe 70 people had come to attend the event. And of those 70 people maybe 20 people hung around to speak with me afterwards. It was just 20 people. Sure. But at the time, having 20 people hang around to talk with me about this subject was 20 more people than I'd previously had to talk about this subject. And so I was THRILLED to say the least.

Some questions were expected. Some not. Either way... throughout all of the time I'd spent writing and editing *Autism On Acid*, I never imagined that anyone would actually take any of this very seriously. I figured that I'd write my book, tell my story, and people would be like "Wow what a strange story about an autistic getting high. Moving on." But that's not how it went. People were interested. People were curious. And somehow or another — despite having spent nearly six years' worth of mornings reading the exact same keyword-specific Google Scholar email alert digests all the way up until the night of that Aware Project presentation — I was still interested, too!

Receiving the support of everyone in that room that night was absolutely everything I needed. Indeed. Because the support of all of those kind and curious strangers allowed me to feel far less alone and also — perhaps most critically of all — relieved to know that this precious and delicate treasure I'd been carrying inside of me for so long could finally be set down and held up and analyzed and considered by more than just me. And I think I feel that same joy right now, editing this current book, knowing that others will be able to feel that same simultaneous blend of relief, support, and validation.

I felt supported that night. Sure. But as time went on after that September presentation, I once again found myself slipping back into a state of self-doubt.

I kept checking my inbox, and the Google Doc copy of the book, daily, waiting to hear from someone, anyone — even if only through a YouTube comment — so that I could progress my understanding.

But once again a lull came about.

A few weeks went by. And yes, I felt some sense of relief as a result of having released my personal truths into the world. Sure. But I was still battling the return of this sense that I was just babbling on about nonsense. And so I fought off this feeling by resuming an ongoing dialogue with my parents; a dialogue that I had already been so fortunate to have been able to revisit, every so often, all throughout all of those years of self-learning. We talked — or, perhaps more accurately, I talked... for a while... Alright... Maybe a long while... — and after yet another one of my signature infodump monologues, and the minute or two or ten my parents needed to process it all, they did something amazing.

They said, "Ok." They gave me space to speak.

They expressed still yet more serious concern, of course. And we definitely talked in circles many times as I attempted to catch them up on a few more years' worth of research and refinement of my personal understandings. But regardless of all of the challenges inherent in the discussion, my parents remained engaged in the conversation. They listened. They cared. And we went about resuming a temporarily paused but forever-open dialogue that I've been so lucky to be able to maintain with them all throughout my many adventures and misadventures in mental health care. And I've said this many times but I really can't thank them enough for all the listening and reading and learning that they've done. I've handed them probably a dozen or so books ranging from academically dense to psychedelically strange. But both my mom and my dad have done what they can to keep up and understand. They've listened and trusted me while still remaining unafraid to voice concerns as they saw fit. It's been such a loving and open dialogue. And I'm so grateful for this. Always. Wow.

Speaking of gratitude, I would also like to express thanks for one other very important person: an individual who wrote me an email about three months after my presentation for the Aware Project.

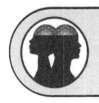 # Klein's Words

December 11, 2019

Hi Aaron,

I received your book yesterday. [...] I wasn't aware of your book and found it only while looking for references on the topic, i.e., Autism and LSD. I was researching those subjects as I'm in the beginning phase of writing a book on my own experience.

It seemed surreal that I found your book, or a book on this topic. I felt that I had to reach out and share a bit of my own experience with LSD. I consider it the most significant event of my life. I was diagnosed with ASD at 40. Two years prior to my diagnosis, I used LSD for the first time. I would learn later it was a significant dose for a first trip :) I experienced ego death. It was spectacular. When I woke the next morning my mind was still. Silent. I would describe to friends that it was as if the volume was muted. The only thoughts I had were those I deliberately held or the present moment, but no longer was there any storm of anxious thoughts. It more or less remains so today. I have vastly more energy than ever before - I attribute this to the reduced mental fatigue once anxious thoughts were gone from my mind. There are many aspects of my life that have been changed by that experience, but most of all self-acceptance. It changed many aspects of my life in a profound way. And it is for that reason, as well as my own perspective of ASD, that I want to write a book as well.

I would be happy to discuss more if you're interested - call or video chat might work best. I look forward to finishing your book.

All The Best,
- Klein

From that point forward, emails and messages and comments began appearing in my notifications and inboxes with gradually increasing frequency — slowly at first, every few weeks; and then, every few days. And now, here in the early months of 2021, there are days in which I get the pleasure and honor of receiving messages from multiple individuals in the span of a single day.

Believe me when I say that I will never, ever tire of hearing these messages and reflections. These words are such treasures to those who share them, and I hope that you, the reader, can also join me in recognizing how special it is to be able to gain a glimpse of the inner worlds of individuals who have navigated such incredibly complex territories all throughout their lives.

2020 Autistic Psychedelic Scrapbook

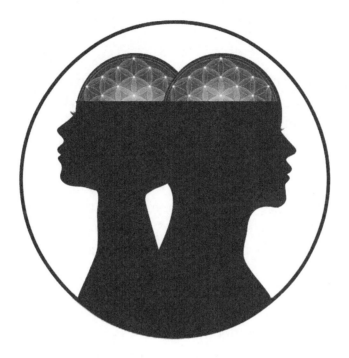

The following section consists of select message exchanges and other related Autistic Psychedelic Community content that came about as a result of the events outlined in "The Story So Far" section of this book. These message excerpts and links to online content are presented so as to establish context and shed light upon the rationale for the formation and continuation of the APC, which has in turn helped to create the core offerings of this book: the personal essays and survey responses.

Throughout this scrapbook section, I will periodically return to narrate/reflect/provide additional context whenever necessary.

To make a clear distinction between my personal narration and the direct quotation of myself or others, I have elected to narrate using this particular font that you're reading right now, in this sentence.

By contrast, this font that you're reading — right now, in this sentence — will be used to indicate any time words have been directly quoted from messages, comments, emails, or other written mediums.

 # Charlie's Words

January 16th, 2020

Hi Aaron,

I just watched a video of your talk for the Aware Project, which I found while researching the effects of LSD on people with ASD. I'm also on the spectrum myself; I was diagnosed with Asperger's at 15 (but disregarded it as an inaccurate diagnosis and didn't fully realize it was correct until just a few months ago), and although it's on the more mild side, it precluded me from feeling empathy, love, and human connection in general. Some years ago, at 26, I got the exact same results from LSD use as you did. I thought it was the craziest thing, couldn't even comprehend what had happened or why, and I couldn't find any other anecdotal evidence of similar occurrences online until very recently, when I found this YouTube video (*viewable via AutisticPsychedelic.com/wiki*).

The way you describe reacting to this podcast was quite literally how I reacted to that guy's account of his experience — understanding empathy within a purely logical framework only to gain emotional awareness from the use of LSD as an adult, and suddenly being able to form what feels like genuine bonds with people, as well as understanding human interaction as a whole — so I guess that makes at least 4 of us? And I suppose there's bound to be more out there. I seriously think we're onto something here with regards to LSD's ability to treat various troubling aspects of ASD.

The reason I decided to contact you is that we're clearly a very small and select group of people. This has been the weirdest, yet most rewarding and life changing thing I've ever experienced, and it's really great to have finally encountered others who can relate. For a while I thought mine was such a marginal case that no one would ever truly understand. So if you're interested, I'd love to hear more about the psychological and emotional changes you've incurred, and I'd be happy to share more of mine. Maybe we can compare notes and somehow build a stronger case for the use of psychedelics as a pharmacological option in the mitigation of ASD-related issues and difficulties.

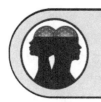

Edwin's Words

January 23rd, 2020

Hi Aaron,

I've just finished listening to the podcast in which you describe your experience of ASD before and after taking LSD. I was literally jumping up and down saying "That was me!" […] Your phraseology encapsulated my feelings of struggling with social situations perfectly. That whole feeling of surviving a social gathering rather than enjoying it.

I was never formally diagnosed with Asperger's, but when some years ago my wife discussed the possibility that I had it with me it just seemed to fit. Until then I could never understand why parties were such a chore, I always made excuses to myself, I assumed that I was having a bad day, that I had drunk too little/too much, the next time would be better. But it never was.

After I considered the possibility of being an Aspie life became a lot simpler, there was nothing I could do to prepare for a social event to make it run more smoothly so I could just be myself.

In my case it was an experience with psilocybin truffles that opened up my emotions and showed me an alternative outlook on life. I had become interested in the clinical trials suggesting the efficacy of psychedelics to treat depression (which I also suffered from intermittently) and three years ago I participated in two ayahuasca ceremonies which certainly alleviated my symptoms of depression, albeit only for a month or so, and also gave me insights suggesting that I needed to go deeper into the psychedelic experience.

After the ayahuasca ceremonies I started microdosing LSD under the protocols established by Jim Fadiman & for a while this helped me with my low moods & made me more open.

Then last year I heard about the psychedelic retreats […] held in Holland where the truffles were legal. I decided to sign up for a 4 day retreat in September. I had a lot of misgivings because the retreats were attended by up to 16 people and of course being isolated with 16 strangers for 4 days is not something an Aspie is going to be happy about! In the event the retreat went perfectly, I gained more from it than I could have possibly imagined. My 'intentions' were to be more loving and open with other people, especially with my wife; to try and be the best version of myself.

What happened during the psilocybin trip was transformational, I felt as if my outer shell that trapped my emotions inside and prevented others from reaching me was ripped open. I was overwhelmed by unconditional love for everyone around me and wanted to care for them and protect them. When I returned home the feeling of love persisted although it was largely directed at my wife (she didn't complain!) but for once I sought out encounters with neighbours and even strangers.

Prior to the psilocybin trip I would have avoided meeting neighbours in the driveway because I'd run out of things to say after 'hi'. My wife could spend 30 minutes happily chatting over the fence and I'd be like 'but what could you possibly say that would take 30 minutes?' Now I knew! On one occasion she came home to find me in the front garden chatting to a scaffolder who had come to remove scaffolding from the front of our house. Previously I would have stayed indoors until he left, or awkwardly talked about the weather, now I was 'chatting', about what I can't remember, but it just flowed.

In addition to being better able to relate to individuals, I experienced a further sea change in my behaviour. Previously I had shied away from any group activities, I had private yoga and tai chi lessons and could not imagine attending a class with others. Immediately after the psychedelic experience I cancelled my one-on-one classes and started attending group sessions. Furthermore I sought out group experiences, large and small. Within a couple of months I had attended a five rhythms dance event with cacao ceremony, A Wim Hof method workshop and a kundalini yoga retreat.

All of these events were quite intimate and involved a lot of one-on-one work within a group setting. Six months ago you couldn't have paid me to attend, now I was paying to attend!

My transition is not as complete as yours appears to be, I am still not great in social gatherings and I find small talk difficult, but your experience has given me hope that the judicious use of psychedelics can give me the direct emotional contact with everyone at large that I am now enjoying with my wife and close friends.

Thank you for your courage in making your experiences public!
Edwin

January 26th, 2020 — Email Response to Edwin

Hi Edwin,

Awesome!

Also, I wanted to say that for all of the emails I've received now like this, yours is among the nearest to overlapping so much with my own story. Most especially the switch from being more inclined to isolating versus seeking social encounters. I'm always still learning, and I value my introvertedness now more than ever. But the world def requires us to be social extroverts at times, and I'm glad to have skills on that end also. Or rather, a means to have the skills. […]

Could you share a bit about the psilocybin retreat? And how that contrasted your experiences with LSD and Ayahuasca?

With Gratitude
-Aaron

January 26th, 2020 — Email from Edwin

Hi Aaron,

I share your feelings on the value of introvertedness and being able to 'turn on' the social skills. I think for me it is about having the choice now. I'll never be a social butterfly or conversational ringleader but at least now I feel more able to hold my own in social settings without it being a chore.[…]

Although I had dabbled with LSD and psilocybin in my student days (back in the 70's, I am a sixty something!) I had only ever taken it recreationally. I had heard of the Ayahuasca ceremonies that took place in Goa […] but had never really been that interested as the idea of 'purging' put me off. […] Three years ago my yoga teacher mentioned that she had attended a ceremony and I was eager to hear the details and on the basis of her account I decided that I would attend the next ceremony. I Googled 'Ayahuasca ceremony' endlessly to try and prepare myself but nothing can prepare you for the event of course.

The first ceremony taught me that preparation, intention and integration are as important as the psychedelic experience itself. I had an interesting experience but the message that came over was 'you have not prepared properly so you are not going to receive the wisdom you expect' I was basically shown a part of myself that I had to acknowledge and address before I was going to get any revelations or deep insights. That in itself was a revelation and it did put me on a path to resolve the issue.

The psilocybin retreat was a joy from start to finish. The facilitators came from different backgrounds, a mixture of clinical psychologists and new age shamen. They used various techniques to build a bond of trust between themselves and the participants, such as circle work, dance, tai chi and yoga. Most of the participants had never had any experience with psychedelics and were naturally quite nervous about the actual 'trip', but the lead facilitator was an expert in visualisation techniques and she ensured that everyone had a gentle and positive experience. The trip itself was taken lying down, listening to music with eye shades.

After the trip we were encouraged to take a silent walk in the woods surrounding the retreat, accompanied by a facilitator (who remained sober throughout). As to my own experiences, they were truly transformational. As I mentioned before, I had set intentions of being more open and loving but I was also looking for answers to my next phase of life as I was in the process of retiring and selling my business and feeling very unsure about how my future would pan out. Without writing a trip report, which I know from experience is usually as interesting as listening to someone describing a dream they had, I will just say that I got everything I wanted from the experience plus a whole lot more.

One of the things that the facilitators ask you in the one-to-one before taking the psilocybin is whether you are OK with physical contact (as in having your hand held or maybe an arm around the shoulder if you appear to be distressed or in need of comfort) I had said I didn't really have a problem with that but they shouldn't expect me to initiate it. In the event, at the peak of the session I was hugging one facilitator and crying with no shame or embarrassment whilst proclaiming that this was the most beautiful thing that had happened to me and that I had been reborn, I had discovered my inner warrior!

The issues that had blocked my first Ayahuasca experience just disappeared and I understood they were now dealt with and would no longer bother me (they haven't). Whereas with the Ayahuasca ceremony there was no integration afterwards — you basically got yourself together and went home to think about what had just happened, on the retreat there was a whole day and a half to make sense of it, with further group sessions, discussions and another one-to one with a facilitator.

I started keeping a journal afterwards, which has been very useful as it enabled me to monitor my emotions and interactions accurately. So, for around a week I experienced an afterglow such that I almost felt like I was an enlightened being! This gradually faded to a more normal state (but still very positive and outgoing) and after six weeks I had my first setback with a mini meltdown. This was followed by a few weeks where I questioned the validity of the experience and went back to microdosing LSD (which I had given up before the retreat) to raise my mood.

It was shortly after this that I took part in a dance and cacao ceremony and that improved my mood noticeably. A couple of weeks later I went on a kundalini yoga retreat with my yoga teacher and this elevated my mood and social interaction such that once again stopped microdosing, and this is where I am now, almost five months after the psilocybin experience.

For me the effect on my social interactions or reducing my Aspie tendencies is only one part of a much broader range of positive benefits from taking psilocybin. I have got rid of various annoying habits and repetitive thought patterns like the need to over-plan simple events such as meeting someone for lunch. Whereas before I would sit down for days checking Google maps for the best route and finding out where I could park, now I would just take a quick look and jump in the car and drive.

My interests have broadened, I have taken up meditation and my reading choices have expanded to include philosophy and spirituality (before I was purely a science geek) so I feel like I am a more complete and expansive person (if that makes sense). These changes don't seem forced and I don't feel that this is what I should be doing, rather this is now what I want to be doing.

My only recent experiences with LSD have been microdosing. It was a generally positive experience, especially in the early days. I became very motivated and took a keen interest in cooking, creating elaborate meals for my wife each evening. I took an interest in nature and enjoyed long walks in the countryside. As my main reason for microdosing was to alleviate symptoms of depression I have to say it worked well. However, when I was microdosing I wasn't sure when I should stop, it seemed that if I was getting benefits I should just continue, why risk going back to depression? I did take breaks but only for a few weeks at a time. However after the psilocybin retreat I just felt no need to continue, it just didn't seem relevant. I got the same feeling after my yoga retreat, it was as if a part of my brain reconnected with the state it was in during the trip and I was raised to a new level.

I know that the process is a journey, there is no cure, but it is a journey I am enjoying and will continue.
    – Edwin

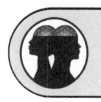

Taylor's Words

February 2nd, 2020

Hi Aaron,

Just listened to your interview on this podcast. I really appreciate you being brave enough to share your story -- and to tell it so well. I'm also on the spectrum, self-diagnosed Aspergers, and use both mushrooms (micro- and low-moderate doses so far) and especially cannabis to self-medicate during the daytime with great results, and I can strongly relate to a lot of what you say about the autistic experience as well as the benefits of the psychedelic experience (though I must admit I haven't yet had as "complete" a trip as you described).

Anyway, I hope you have, but in case you haven't, you truly have to read Switched On by John Elder Robison. The after-effects of your first trip as you described them are very similar to what Elder Robison achieved through his own, vastly different form of treatment.

Reading his book a number of years ago introduced me to Aspergers and changed my life; even his interview on Fresh Air (*viewable via AutisticPsychedelic.com/wiki*) brought me to tears.

Your speaking out is sure to change many lives as well.

-Taylor

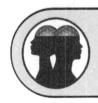

Riley's Words

Feb. 21st, 2020

Dear Aaron Paul,

I just saw your talk at the Aware Project on Youtube and I am very thankful for it. [...]

Just a couple of days ago I realized that I might be on the autistic spectrum through coincidentally watching another video about autism. It was an almost revelatory moment. All of the sudden the unconnected dots that made up my life so far connected and made up a picture of who I really am. I am not diagnosed yet, but I feel like everything is falling into place. There are so many symptoms that people with [autism spectrum disorder] describe that I can relate to, and that have caused problems as well as greatness in my life, that it would seem ridiculous to ignore it from now. It's like a path finally opened that I can and want to walk down now.

I have been using psychedelics since about 2 and a half [years] for a self-healing process. This was obviously before my realization that I might be on the autistic spectrum. So there was no specific intention to direct the psychedelic experience towards [autism spectrum disorder]. However it became clear very early on that this might help me more than other people and I can totally relate to a lot of things you are describing in your talk. I believe that my position on the spectrum might be more that of a tendency than a full-blown syndrome and I am definitely high-functioning. But all this really is up to exploration for me now as it is brand new.

Anyway, I can relate so much to what you are talking about!

The way you describes what your life felt like before, what psychedelics do to you, and what happened to you afterwards is very much what happened to me, although it was a lot less conscious in my case, because i kind of stumbled into the psychedelic experience in first place and didn't prepare myself as well as you did.

Please let me know whether I can be of any help in raising more attention to this subject!

Feb 21st, 2020 — Email to Riley

Hi,

Thank you so much for your email. I never tire of receiving these types of messages. And it seems the world is full of people like us. So the good news is that we're not alone in our stumbling across this phenomenon :)

It's funny you asked about sharing your story because I'm in the midst of gathering stories like these for the purpose of serving as a precursor to research into this space and also generally helping one another and others like this understand this phenomenon [...]

Thanks again for reaching out. You and I and others like us may have stumbled across something very helpful for the world :)

With Gratitude,
Aaron Paul Orsini

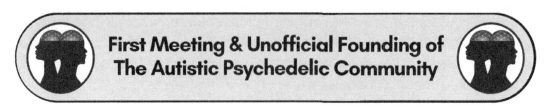

First Meeting & Unofficial Founding of The Autistic Psychedelic Community

— *March 29th, 2020* —

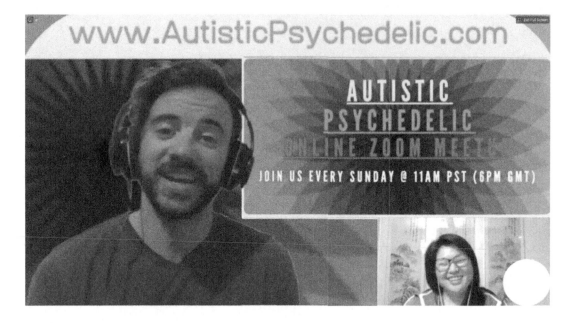

Once upon a Sunday in the middle of the beginning of a pandemic, the Autistic Psychedelic Community held its first meeting. Justine and I created a small meetup invite & posted it on a few psychedelic community calendars. About a dozen people came. And we all seemed to be mutually excited to have the chance to speak with one another about these topics.

We have been gathering weekly via Zoom, every Sunday, ever since. And we're now up to a few hundred members between our various social media groups. Our open Zoom meetings exist as an accepting space for those looking to share personal truths and learn from the personal truths and views shared by others in a collaborative, peer-supported setting.

We welcome all neurotypes.
Join us anytime @
www.AutisticPsychedelic.com

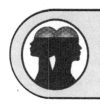

Stefan's Words

April 3rd, 2020

Hi Aaron, my name is Stefan, I am in my thirties and I am from Germany. I read your excellent book and could relate to many things you wrote about, because just one year ago I had my first LSD-trip and for the first time some things became clear and intuitive to me.

But let me tell you about my backstory first: My whole life I knew something is "not right" with me. I never was able to truly connect with anybody. I was only able to talk about facts. Communication for me was just an exchange of information (I send information, I receive information) – nothing more. Questions like "Hey, what's up?" or "How are you?" resulted in an error in my brain (because that was no information) and with time I learned to just say a memorized sentence, without any emotion, just for the sake of an acceptable answer. As a child I already realized that people find me weird, some were even bullying me, and always wondered why, because it didn't make any sense: I was always friendly, was good in school and never was a bully etc.

I was always very good at math and logical thinking but in my puberty this wasn't enough anymore to be accepted in my class. I instinctively knew that "normal kids" had some kind of special connection with each other and could sense their emotions and intuitions but never could understand how they do this. I thought, maybe I just need more time to develop – that I am just a "late- bloomer" and my time will finally come to have some cool friends and a girlfriend. But in my 20s I realized that something was "not OK" with me.

While studying at the university I was mostly alone. To work with new groups of people was a nightmare, and sometimes I am wondering today how I managed to accomplish all this…

I was researching a lot on the internet. Finally, after years of reading about depression, autism, personality disorders etc. I was 99% sure that I am autistic because the more I read about this condition, the more sense my whole life made to me (I was also diagnosed with ADHD when I was 10 and again when I was 31 – my official autism-diagnosis is still pending...).

Now to the "good part": 2 years ago I ordered LSD and started microdosing which helped me a bit. My mind was clearer and I could talk better, my voice was stronger. But sometimes it didn't work and I had kind of a blurry view and was irritated by mediocre things. So it was a fifty-fifty-chance if it works or not.

After 1 year I had the courage to finally try a big dose. And it was a very good trip! I was with my mother and brother and during the trip I started to realize some things. I felt that energy, which I called "wave", this was the natural way life formed itself. And I also could identify when this wave was not there – when the situation was artificial and not natural. For example: My brother saw me and was making fun of me when he realized that I was tripping. But I immediately realized that this was only his brain making fun of me (because he used logic to make a bad joke) and I felt that this isn't real, I said to him, "This is not the wave, this was like a hard edge for me" – it was not good. While talking to them I realized how much their brain got in the way and blocked the "wave". I tried to explain to them that all is natural and they laughed because they (or: their logical brain) couldn't make any sense of what I was saying. I then realized that all problems stem from the fact, that people have their brain "in their way" which doesn't allow the flow, or the wave, to form.

I then talked to my mother and explained that if any mentally ill person was in that state I was in then their anxiety-disorder or PTSD or whatever would instantly dissolve, because these things only existed in the brain, which aren't real – because there is ONLY energy, the wave.

This realization was very extreme and it suddenly was so easy. I also could watch them in the eyes without feeling discomfort.

The days after the first trip ended, I realized that I had some permanent changes (until today): For whatever reason my stamina got better. I could run farther than the week before and going up some stairs didn't make me as exhausted as before – weird (This is no placebo btw because I surely didn't expect that, but after the first 4 stairs I must go up to my home I thought "hm.. my breath is absolutely calm and normal, strange...") But the best thing is: I am not getting a meltdown anymore, when I hear sudden loud noises.

Before, when I heard a dog barking outside or a loud car or a door slammed or someone dropped a plate, I was getting very angry, almost raging – especially if I tried to concentrate. This is 100% gone.

Today when there is a loud noise anywhere it doesn't "hurt" anymore, I am totally calm. This second example is a proof that something MUST have changed in my brain. The sensory input got better, my synapses can handle loud noises much, much better.

One bitter-sweet thing with the LSD-trips is that as you come down from the high, you slowly realize that the effects are gone and that the autistic mind takes over again. But the insights I got will stay with me forever.

Final words: LSD for me was a wonderful experience. I got to know the energy, the wave, that is out there, that helps people to bond with each other. It always has to be natural and easy – I could feel, what it was like, to be neurotypical. But sadly LSD also showed me that I have a "defect" brain, that I just couldn't get in this state while sober, because the logical part of my brain is WAY too strong. Also my emotions were not activated, I still feel very numb, as if I am dreaming my life.

Just like you Aaron, I think there must be much more research. We have to know what brain regions are involved in autism and how we can manipulate them for therapeutic use. But one thing makes me very hopeful: The fact that my brain was ABLE to experience this natural energy, without having the logical brain in the way. That means that I have the right synapses, but they are just wrongly programmed. I really hope psychedelics will be reclassified so that at least the researchers can make fast progress.
Greetings from Germany, - Stefan

APC's Neurodiverse Neuroscience With Psychedelic Researcher Dr. Katrin Preller

— May 3rd, 2020 —

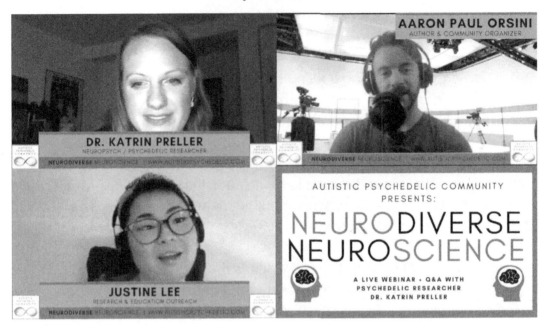

In May, 2020, Justine and I were honored to host a one-hour interview and open community Q+A with Swiss psychedelic researcher, Dr. Katrin Preller (M.Sc., Neuropsychology and Clinical Psychology, University of Konstanz; PhD, Department of Psychiatry, Psychotherapy, and Psychosomatics, University of Zurich). During our conversation, we discussed Dr. Preller's most recent research exploring the measurable effects of psychedelics such as LSD and psilocybin on aspects of social cognition.

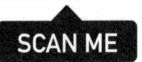

SCAN ME

 Visit AutisticPsychedelic.com/video or Scan QR Code on This Page to Watch

WHAT DO YOU WANT TO TELL THE WORLD ABOUT PSYCHEDELICS & AUTISM?

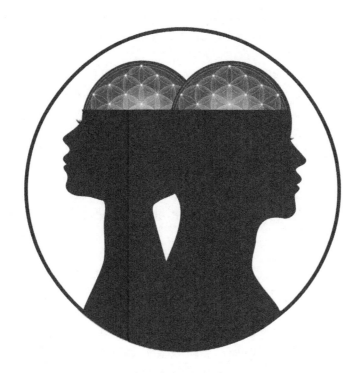

PERSONAL ESSAYS FROM

THE AUTISTIC PSYCHEDELIC COMMUNITY

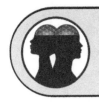 # Sabrina's Words

Content Warning: Discussion of Abuse

My name is Sabrina.

I'm a 36 year-old autistic woman born and raised in Mexico.

As a child, I got beaten up by my parents every time I behaved "weird, antisocial, disrespectful or defiant." I soon learned not to move, not to talk, and to avoid as much as possible getting in "trouble."

I also had extreme difficulty making friends and keeping them. I wanted to fit in with all my heart. I fell asleep countless nights wondering what was wrong with me, why nobody liked me. I pretended to be happy, but I was miserable.

As a woman, I experienced abuse in every single form possible from romantic relationships. I accepted all because I was afraid of losing the only "connections" and "love" I finally had.

After years of trauma and abuse, I experienced the most intense burnout of my life. I was bouncing from episodes of emotional numbness to outbursts of sadness or anger. I was unable to talk as eloquently as I did before. I had an increased sensitivity to sensory input and extreme difficulty with changes. I was in a dark place.

I learned about psychedelics after reading a scientific study about them and their efficacy in treating depression and anxiety. It took me two years to take them.

Psychedelics are life-changing, but they are POTENT; they are both challenging and healing. These substances should be taken with responsibility, and every person must do their due diligence about the specific psychedelic substance/plant they would like to use, the setting where they will be taken, making sure the sitter/shaman/facilitator is someone that can stay calm during difficult situations, and also someone who is knowledgeable, trustworthy, responsible, and caring.

During and right after taking psychedelics, some moments were confusing, fearful, or sad. But many were joyous, connected, loving, and ineffable. That's why Integration is the MOST critical part of the healing.

Integration is what happens after a ceremony/trip; it's what you make of the teachings, messages, and insights that you get from psychedelics, and the changes you make in your life consistent with those lessons.

Psychedelics helped me with my depression, anxiety, PTSD, and to accept and love all of me. Thanks to psychedelics, I could forgive everyone who hurt me; I realized that hurt people hurt people, and psychedelics helped me break that cycle. They showed me boundaries are an essential part of forgiveness. I was able to let my suffering go; I was not a captive of it anymore.

I learned to love my uniqueness, my solitude, and my bluntness. I stopped wishing to be someone else; I embraced everything I am. I realized there is absolutely nothing wrong with me; there never was.

Lastly, I would like to emphasize that psychedelics are not "miraculous"; they aren't a "cure"; they are a tool to improve your life.

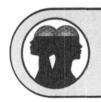 # Bobby's Words

Content Warning: Discussion of Suicidal Ideation

Psychedelic drugs irreversibly changed my life.

I was 22 when I had my first psychedelic experience. I had spent most of my life being scared of illegal drugs because of fears of addiction & overdosing. But after a downward spiral into depression and being on the borderline of suicide, suddenly the potential consequences of these drugs didn't seem so bad. I had been inspired by the Beatles, Steve Jobs, and neuroscientist Sam Harris into believing that psychedelic drugs could be an answer to my imprisoned state of mind, and it now seems all of these inspirational figures were right. However, nothing could have prepared me for the experience itself and no words I write could fully describe it — but nonetheless I will try.

I took my first dose of LSD in my flat with a school friend, and what started as a laid-back time watching TV and listening to music quickly spiralled into internal chaos. I began to feel as if I were losing my sense of self and that as far as I knew that would be it — I was going to die. I did not feel any physical pain besides panic but the voice in my head that is always there was being stripped away, and this was terrifying. As I'm writing this it doesn't feel so serious, but to give you a window into my mindset at the time, I was verbally shouting "I am a person" because it no longer felt true and I didn't want to forget it. I tried to call my mom to say goodbye, but the phone may as well have been an alien technology.

All of this seemed traumatic in the moment — that is at least until I suddenly accepted that my life as "me" was over. And *that's* when all of the panic and negativity dissipated. To describe this in a different way I have some analogies: while you go through life, you're a leaf on a branch on a tree. Well during this moment I was the entire tree; thus all of the branches and leaves of The Tree were also me. Suddenly the entire universe made sense and I was experiencing time, reality, and the universe objectively instead of subjectively. From this vantage point, it seems as if anything is possible.

Once this state began to subside, I started to be "me" again, but something was different. I "felt" different. I don't mean that I was in a new headspace. I mean I literally perceived reality differently. I could feel how others felt and this was new. I don't believe I lacked empathy before this experience because I could always analyze how people felt. But I had never been able to "feel" it. Suddenly so many things I'd never understood nor experienced before were now seemingly available to me. I then began to cry hysterically. It was as if I had new eyes; as if a filter system had been turned off.

That day in 2017 marked the start of my journey with psychedelics and my life has since tended in the right direction. Since my first trip, I have experimented with both microdosing and macrodosing and both approaches have personally helped me tremendously. Although I would say my first experience was the most traumatic of them all, it was also the most powerful and defining one as well.

Although I wish that I could say that my story continued happily ever after all of this, unfortunately it is not so simple. In the years since my first experience, the "new me" sometimes began to fade again — although never fading so much so as to resemble the person I'd been before the first experience. Likewise, the world at times has been difficult to exist within. Even so, I felt I gained a tool with psychedelics. And I felt that I could use this tool to solve things and get back to a place of happiness.

To use another analogy: imagine that happiness is achieved by driving a car at a constant speed. When my car starts to jerk & slow down sometimes, I might struggle to return to the speed of happiness. But psychedelics are like a jump start to get back to "normality"; they help me understand why things slowed down in the first place. In this way, psychedelics are *a tool to find* contentedness but not *a replacement for* the contentedness itself.

I know my default mode network is very logical and often robotic but these drugs helped me to cultivate a self that is more likeable, compassionate, confident, motivated, creative, content, moral and loving. I owe my life to these drugs. And because of my experiences with psychedelics, I am a happier person and to me that is why we are all here: to share this experience together, to grow, to love.

I foresee a future in which psychedelics can be used legally worldwide to treat both depression and the more troublesome aspects of the autistic experience. Similarly, in light of all of this, I also foresee a future that is a happier one for the whole of humanity.

Jay's Words

Psychedelics are a special interest of mine. Until my early twenties, I was quite "left-brained": an analytical, somewhat sheltered, straight "A" student. My experiences with psychedelics, especially DMT and psilocybin, opened me up to an entirely new understanding of consciousness. The world became pregnant with magic, energy, synchronicity, and emotion. I felt the power of my own neural networks becoming connected and integrated in new ways.

My journey with psychedelics has not been an easy one. Many people share that they feel more connected with others after taking these substances; for me, the opposite has been true. In the early years of my life, I passed as neurotypical and, while introverted and easily overwhelmed, had a fairly typical relationship pattern. After using psychedelics, I became more acutely aware of my neurodivergence. I have become increasingly selective when it comes to friendships; unless I feel a genuine intellectual and energetic connection with someone, I would rather spend time alone.

During my psychedelic journeys, I feel intimately in touch with the presence of the Other – a higher intelligence with a very alien quality. Because of my tendency toward obsession, I have at times become ungrounded in my quest to understand this force. What is it, and how does it work? Is it simply an unfamiliar part of my unconscious mind, or have I wandered into another frequency of reality, populated with entities – or is this an artificial distinction created by the illusion of self?

I would rather live an interesting life than a simple one, and that is what psychedelics have enabled me to do. Rather than follow the linear life course I had originally envisioned, my path has been winding and beautiful. I have found a profession well-suited to my strengths and quirks. I have found soul connection in a partner much older than I am. I have found companionship in those willing to delve into the secrets of the universe. And in moments of isolation, I have found solace and adventure in the mysteries of my own mind.

I believe psychedelics should be legalized not because they are inherently safe or healing, but because it is a human right to explore the frontiers of consciousness. I assume personal risk every time I drive a car; there is a chance I will get lost, injured, or even die. All of this is worthwhile, though, because modern transportation makes my world so much bigger. Psychedelics are the same. I deserve autonomy to experience good and bad trips, freedom to get lost from time to time, and trust in my ability to command my own mind. As do you; as does everyone.

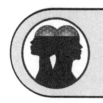 # Shae's Words

I'm a 27-year-old cis woman living in the United States, and this year I was diagnosed with autism spectrum disorder.

Growing Up Autistic

Because I easily excelled in school and did not have behavior problems — two primary points of intervention — my neurodivergence went largely unnoticed by adults. My mother knew that I was similar to her, but many years would pass before her and I would have the language to describe it exactly.

As a child, I was socially awkward and often completely unaware of my awkwardness. I frequently made missteps or disrupted social situations. And eventually, a primary coping mechanism developed: I would freeze, and do nothing in order to avoid doing something wrong or breaking some social rule that no one would tell me about.

In addition to this "freeze" response, I also had a tendency toward meltdowns. Nowadays, because of my awareness of my autism, it's apparent that these meltdowns in my younger years were often a result of my sensory sensitivities (especially those related to sound, temperature, and new people).

In the years leading up to high school, I went through phases of various special interests until I found my true hyperfocus: how to change the world. I watched as the connective nature of the Internet empowered an entire generation to challenge oppressive systems, and this awareness imprinted upon me the unshakeable belief that we *can* change the world.

During undergraduate schooling, I studied social movement history and theory, and chose my major with the intention of helping to change our minds so that we can change our systems. My entire identity is enmeshed with this work, and I can't imagine doing anything else.

All throughout my life, verbal communication has always been difficult for me. A combination of pragmatic language difficulties and delayed auditory processing make it difficult (and sometimes impossible) for me to meaningfully participate in verbal conversations. I also do not think in words. I think in colors, shapes, and sound, which I then translate into words. This translation is a time-consuming process that makes verbal communication very inefficient for me. Thankfully, written communication is less energy intensive, and therefore much more comfortable.

My Autistic Psychedelic Emergence

When I was 18 years old, my relationship with psychedelics began with a subthreshold dose of DMT. This experience allowed me to see/hear what I now know to be my innate synesthesia — a blend of color and sound that dissolves language. After this DMT experience came experiences with mushrooms, then LSD, then MDMA, then MDA, then ketamine.

MDMA

My first experience with MDMA resulted in my first-ever experience of effortless and fluid verbal communication. Normally, my verbal processing felt like crossing the chasm between synesthesia and words using spaced-out stepping stones. But when I took MDMA, it felt as though a bridge directly translating synesthesia into language was formed. This change lasted for up to three days after taking MDMA, but was always temporary.

LSD

A series of regular LSD doses — some of which were taken in combination with MDMA or MDA — effectively laid the foundation for me to experience an actual synesthesia-language bridge. The breakthrough happened the first time I took a relatively high dose of LSD. Although I was nonverbal — in the moment, during the peak of this experience — the experience as a whole granted me ongoing access to verbal language in a way that I never dreamed could be real for me. Nowadays, my nonverbal/minimal verbal episodes still occur — especially when I'm anxious, upset, or experiencing sensory overload — but these episodes are no longer my default state.

Microdosing LSD has also played its own unique role in my life. To put it one way, microdosing LSD feels like putting on glasses that simplify sensory information and social interactions in a way that makes some situations much less overwhelming. While microdosing, I am focused, energized, and less anxious, which makes the idea of going out into the world much less intimidating.

Ketamine

Ketamine played a very distinct role in my autistic psychedelic emergence as well. In specific, my use of ketamine has allowed me to suspend my compulsion to attempt to translate my synesthesia into language. By suspending my compulsive engagement in this unconscious form of "cognitive masking" — which ketamine helped to reveal to me as an exhausting aspect of my processing that slows me down a lot — I've been able to experience moments of pure synesthesia that have in turn allowed me to engage in intense informational processing and intense emotional processing.

Ketamine is also the only reason that I have been able to tease apart my sensory experience and identify specific points of distress. Before obtaining these insights, my sensory experience was overwhelming and energy-consuming, but it was often unclear exactly what the problem was at any given moment. In this way, ketamine helped me pull these sensory layers apart so that I could address specific points of discomfort before they escalated into a meltdown or a panic attack.

My Autistic Psychedelic Superpowers

Ten years ago, I never imagined that I would have been able to verbally communicate the way I am able to verbally communicate now. I also have a better understanding of my sensory sensitivities. This journey is ongoing, but I definitely feel like I am currently in an integration phase. Being formally diagnosed has been validating, and I am slowly unmasking and accepting what it is to be a neurodivergent person in a neurotypical world. I do not ever feel disabled by my autism, only by the ableism taught by capitalism and white supremacy.

In summary, psychedelics liberated me from a sensory-processing-related language prison. I would not be able to be the organizer I am today — nor would I hold the intention of serving as a healer in the future — without my relationship with psychedelics. Like Greta Thunberg, I believe that autism can be a superpower, and I am so grateful that I have an opportunity to develop mine.

 # Gregory's Words

Before I was diagnosed with autism, I had no prior knowledge of autism. The only things I knew about autism were the perceptions presented in the media — that an autism diagnosis requires medication or the suppression of personality or that autism is simply not good.

After being diagnosed, however, I suddenly realized that all the reasons I had been bullied, or cast out from groups, or called "weird" — or whatever other words others would choose to make it clear to me that I was 'different' — were not 'my fault'.

In the past, I spent a lot of my life unknowingly 'masking'… I tried to 'solve' social experiences in the same way I might have approached an engineering problem: I analyzed myself, the interactions, and how I might iterate on what happened (what I said, gestures, etc.), and then I'd try again… and repeat ad nauseum. That was my life — that is to say, my life when I had a poor self-image.

But then a psychedelic experience eroded all of that… and exorcised those self-perceptions. I saw myself, my qualities, and my character. And for the first time, I could appreciate who I was, who I've been, *and* who I am.

After this psychedelic experience, I was able to finally connect with my thoughts — and with myself — without experiencing constant worry, self-criticism, and shame. In feeling good about myself, I became more capable of appreciating myself as I am — as colorful, diverse, vibrant … like a spectrum. And I became aware of how the qualities that defined me were simply just unique differences that could be seen as exceptional. Indeed. Autism is exceptional.

As time went on, I became even more proud of who I am. I felt good about myself. And I've been expressing this good feeling through my appearance, my mood, my interactions, and my art. For the first time in a long time, I've been able to feel like I have something to share; something *worth* sharing.

And I now have a deep connection to the process of making art — a process that I gave up long ago because I didn't think I could do it.

As I became more open to sharing about myself and my experiences, I also felt inspired to change the perception about autism. And so I decided to start hosting a local meeting for others who may be on the spectrum.

I continue to host this meeting ongoing, all in an effort to change the perception of autism from something that is seen only as a disability into something that is also seen as exceptional.

I hope that autistics feel proud of who they are. I hope that autistics feel they are not alone in their experience. And I hope that autistics also feel they have remarkable qualities — even if others fail to notice or recognize such qualities — because indeed, autism is exceptional.

In regards to my psychedelic experience, I would say to anyone… don't go looking for that. I feel what made my own experience transformative — and "magical" even — is that I had no prior expectation nor reports to draw from. I essentially went in "blind". I wasn't looking to change… and I believe that this absence of expectation was a key foundation that made the process of change possible.

I didn't think much of it when I said to a friend, "The experience you need to have will find you."

My interpretation (for myself) is that when I have wanted to 'change' an aspect of myself, I sought a specific modality, and set a specific timeline, among other things… all of which made me anxious of my progress or not. The act of trying to set or force expectations upon myself that certain things or results would happen in a rote-like manner has often been a recipe for disappointment.

The most enlightening thing I can offer is that experience comes in many forms, and that the act of being open to the idea that anything can happen is, in its own way, a helpful change to undergo. Although routines and modalities can be beneficial at times, they are not nearly as powerful as the simple belief in myself, and the welcoming of all possibilities that may come.

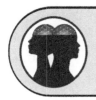

Herald's Words

I have difficulties with the questions and categories presented in the survey so I would like to ignore them and use this text field for a free elaboration of my experiences and thoughts as an autistic who has had psychedelic experiences.

In my life I deal a lot with fundamental questions related to the pressure to perform or the pressure to be productive ("Leistungsdruck" in German). Much of this pressure relates to capitalist ideologies of human worth measured based on the amount that an individual brings into an economy. This particular type of pressure has influenced my experiences a large amount. The experience of shame-free enjoyment has been rare in life but I was able to consciously dive in and out — experiencing/indulging and observing/watching during psychedelic experiences. It was illuminating to be able to control the switching between worlds indeed.

When in a psychedelic state of mind — especially when I have the best setting which I believe includes having all the time in the world so that I can be fully immersed in only the present moment, with no pressure to do anything and no appointments to attend to — then I am free.

In this type of setting, I feel LSD is a plus; a gateway to allowing something. This is how LSD seems to me.

With LSD, I feel things even more intensely. With LSD, I feel in a better "order" and my experience seems less chaotic or blurred or confusing. This clarity in turn leads to (if acted upon logically) taking better care of situations and trusting something that people call intuition which is… something? Nothing? *gestures wildly* haha.

When it comes to planning psychedelic experiences, I think it is important to analyze and take care to imagine and create the best setting for a free deep dive…

No matter where I experience psychedelics, I always like to spend time contemplating/visualizing spiritual metaphors and imageries related to consciousness. E.g. that energy is already there. That energy doesn't really have to be summoned or forced. Instead, that energy comes about as a result of relaxation and release of tension and doubt. When we are free of doubt, we can enjoy movement and creative energy. And we can feel the energy deeply because it is fully available and flowing through us.

I feel it's very very very important to have a good setting (in your life in general, and also during psychedelic trips).

For example: I have the privilege to have very warm and accepting friends and a good social setting in general. The setting greatly impacts my energy levels/emotional state/reactiveness in terms of feeling active or passive or anxious or relaxed. For example: If I know I have a warm nest then I can therefore explore the world bravely. And this is important.

In life and during psychedelic experiences, I require an emotionally very close and warm level of connection but I don't force that. I invite this connection and every boundary is held up on a pedestal in respect and thankfulness. This description may seem to be rigid or an extreme way of thinking but it is important to make sure that everyone is held somehow holy and never shamed, shunned, or talked badly about in life or during psychedelic experiences.

During psychedelic experiences, I think in a very visual way and I just come from the heart. I sometimes enjoy the experience of a very quiet and completely expectation-free place; a place that is reminiscent of where babies would be sleeping.

In life or during psychedelic experiences, sometimes the tension rises and people become angry or begin projecting values on one other. When this happens, something seems to cry out inside of me. When I was younger, I used to shy away from people to protect myself. But now, after psychedelic experiences and also general life experiences, I feel I have more freedom to choose individually and, depending on the situation, I feel more brave and feel I have more inner freedom. I playfully protect everyone who is being gossiped about, saying things like "Oh wait, this same gossip could be said about me. Why are people shaming others for liking something I could also like?" In other words: I try to ruin the social hierarchy games when they appear. And I get more comfortable in that role, being my naive childish self, asking questions without fear of seeming stupid.

Thanks to psychedelics and personal growth, I trust my own moral compass. For example, I know that it is not nice to make fun of someone non-consensually. I know that we can simply answer questions rationally. And because I know these things and have this moral compass, I get to foster shared values in my close social circle.

Even after all of these experiences and opportunities for growth, it is still difficult for me to really deeply vibe and lose myself sometimes. I usually watch and observe situations carefully as they unfold in order to protect myself because I don't usually pick up on hidden intentions otherwise. In an all-autistic group of persons, usually everything can be taken literally without any problems. Autistics can understand one another in a word-for-word sort of way. Autistics can trust processes when the processes are transparent, visible, and consensual, without hierarchy. That's at least what I have determined based on the input of other autistics and the actual connections I have formed.

Some other thoughts I have based on experiences:

I'm super sensitive to morals, ethics, tension, authenticity, feelings like love and loathe in the air, feelings in general, and I feel a conflict with people when they act differently based on who they are interacting with at the time.
I believe I have a good heart but this has made my mother very fearful and protective of me because I give so much love, joy, and trust even when I ought not do this or feel this way.

In my opinion, I can actually be only really authentic if there are no hidden intentions of "using" me. And this makes it extremely hard to navigate among people that tend to be inauthentic or do not seem to have such a strict inner moral compass as I have. Some people seem to exclusively rely on the fear of consequences to guide their actions.

I also have really present difficulties with the normative capitalist concept of labour. I work best when I experience authentic connection and intrinsic (doing things because I want to do them) type of motivation.

This need for authentic, intrinsically valued work makes me a loving helper, because I feel joyful when others are happy, but I also have difficulty with the typical work environments wherein people can be easily exploited. I also have a tendency to appear disrespectful when I prioritize my physical processes (health, nutrition, my body being free of tension). But I do not mean to be disrespectful. I just need to prioritize my physical needs so that I can be fully present for the work in the way I enjoy. Let me repeat this in a different way: I know that if I cannot prioritize my physical needs, I will suffer and feel my health decline because I neglected myself, and my work also will suffer.

Another example of me appearing to be disrespectful is when I am running late even though I have made it transparent beforehand that I would need the extra time. To other people, my delaying makes me appear unreliable. But this is not the case. I can be fully reliable if I am allowed to be REALLY present as I complete the task in a manner that is appropriate for the task. I don't thrive on extrinsic motivational concepts and rewards as these concepts feel empty and depressing. To say this another way: I need to understand the "why" in order to be motivated. This need for a "why" can make me appear stubborn to others. Even so, I know there's a lot of value for all of the workers if this need for knowing "why" is respected.

In my opinion, people seem to not dive that deeply into experiences unless they are very compassionate, open-minded, and aware of other peoples' intuitions, interests, and self-knowledges. I need people to see me on the same level as themselves — and also on the same level as they would see a young person or a very old person or a high-support-needing person or a non-verbally-speaking person or any person because we are all people.

I need people to communicate their own boundaries with a level of mutual respect and compassion. I need people to not start a fight and to not dominate one another because I cannot shut off my inner compass. I am so sensitive to it that I become empty and noncommunicating and depressed and tense at times. My sensitive moral compass makes me feel fearful of the world and at the same time numb and as though I will implode. And because I tend to go down exactly that spiral, I often remain highly misunderstood.

If I have the right communicative setting, I am able to be a very healing presence, and this has been told to me a lot of times by people close to me. When they tell me that I am a healing presence, I am filled with lots of joy — so much joy that I could really just explode (in a good way!) thinking about it. Over time, I have gained the privilege to let out my healing presence but I still shy away often when there is hierarchy and gossip. Related to this: sometimes I hate being perceived and defined because I feel that my physical form seems to just be a container or a medium. My body seems like something like a robot but it is also organic and lovable. Even so, I don't want any form to define me. And that is why I love wearing actual masks (not speaking in metaphors) and also trying to appear "invisible" at times.

I feel that the act of moving the body is a fun experiment that can test one's own focus. Sometimes I move my body just to improve focus. I play around. I dance. I take my mind for a walk. But still, when I'm walking around, I feel that my body is not an "it". I feel that my body is not a noun if this makes sense. In other words: I feel that this body is just an instrument of potentiality. I feel that outer appearances do not need to be judged.

To explain more about this, I will provide some examples:

I love wearing comfortable clothing and also the same clothing that already has holes in the knees or elbows. I enjoy the experience of wearing well-worn clothes, but it's sometimes hard for me to do this because people associate certain judgements with certain outward appearances. Also, as another example: I love the pajama party atmosphere and would love to have exactly that just everywhere. Because an environment that is free of expectation means that people can just hang around and be cozy and jump around excitedly, climbing on things, and taking a nap somewhere just because they feel safe and free of judgement.

In my opinion, environments that are free of judgement are the best environments for me (with or without psychedelics!) because these are the environments in which everyone can feel safe; environments in which people can just be deeply compassionate and caring. In these safe environments, no one is forcing anyone else to do anything. In these safe environments, people help each other freely because they enjoy it. They help each other because everyone benefits from helping others. They help each other because everyone benefits from being helped by others.

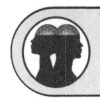

Angel's Words

I'll start at the beginning of my life....Easter, a few years ago....

A vortex of raw energy fell into my world....swirling me deeply into a swim for my life....a dangerous, dark relationship entered ..... I found solid support from a friend who seemed to know .....the friend had a darkness, also, however... I connected with him in a way I rarely experienced.....he showed me familiar traits....as if I were looking at myself.....I asked around...."What is this guy about? He seems to almost be other worldly.....and he really gets angry when you question his behavior.... "Asperger's", an intuitive friend spoke....thus began my journey into the research.... and discovering.....Lo and Behold...Me....I wept for days.....I stood in the middle of my room in a state of pure ecstasy and shouting to the Heavens and Hells of my life........ "I AM NOT BROKEN!!!"

During this same time.... I began micro-dosing psilocybin....I do not remember which came first...autism or psychedelics.....as I said... there was a vortex of energy.....the dark, dangerous man was gone.....I knew who I was... and now ....with the mushrooms....there was more and more of me coming out....and I was beautiful.....my body had a little trouble handling it all..... I was evolving pretty fast.....consciousness rising......

Over the past two years or so....I was always saying..."Oh, that's why I do things this way." or "My, the world is so pretty today..." or..."You know, real connections are rare and I like it that way."...and it goes on......"Oh Goodness, how many doors can I open now.....do I have enough energy for all of this new life?"........."Look at the folks who call me their friend, now....I am really flying high." I still have friends in low places....they keep me real.....

A wonderful metaphysician did a reading for me about 5 years ago....he said, "at age 76....no more troubles"....I'm 78 now....I do believe he got it right...

Now if you want to know about the 76 years before autism and psychedelics.... I guess you will have to wait for the book... however, here is a stream of consciousness riff......

Running, running, running....don't slow me down....the sparkles in the trees and streams are my friends...they talk to me......the animals on the farm need my touch...the flowers so bright on the mud pies I bake for mother....ecstasy flows each day....then it shows me the pain and suffering...of others...."Over here....come into the light...I will help you........I will help you....I will help you....." Love poured from me..... poured..poured....pearls all over the swine....running, running, running.....red shoes dancing....laughing out loud....red lips...tears dried....sullen anger sat quietly....I stopped talking.... afraid if I opened my mouth all holy hell would pour out....no conflict....no conflict...no conflict....bartender was my role....the observer....years...15 cities...100 places...the mask grew thick....then I stopped....the healing began....35 years pulling back the onion skins.....this onion is thick....heavy...crusty....on my knees each day.... cleaning.... cleaning... cleaning.... praying for the ecstasy once again..... and redemption…

So Be It...

Fred's Words

I was diagnosed with depression at a very early age and for a long time I struggled to find a medication that helped with this. I've had depression for so long that I almost forgot what it was like to not have to struggle to find motivation and enthusiasm. But then I started using LSD microdoses with great success. And now, thanks to LSD, I can access the parts of myself that had withered under depression.

LSD does what antidepressants claim to – it reduces the intensity of negative emotions. But it also does what no antidepressant has ever achieved – it enhances positive emotions. Unlike when I took serotonin reuptake inhibitors (SSRIs), I've experienced no negative side effects with LSD, especially in the microdosing range. After looking at the molecular structure and effects of LSD, I've come to think of it as a synthetic serotonin.

Antidepressants are well known for creating dependencies. LSD on the other hand, is non-addictive. Actually no, it would be more accurate to say that it is ANTI-addictive. Studies have shown that it can help people get off of other addictions. But LSD is not a replacement addiction. It has little to no effect when taken two days in a row. And I often find myself forgetting, or just feeling like I don't need to take it on the days I had planned to take it. And that's fine because unlike SSRI's, I don't experience LSD withdrawal.

Throughout my life, I've never had much interest in drugs. I don't even drink. For a long time, I passed on trying any drug and said it was because I didn't want my experiences to be dulled, or my personality to be altered. But in contrast to many drugs, LSD actually enhances the senses – it opens me up by turning down filters in the brain that prevent me from experiencing the world as I once did, when I experienced certain things for the very first time.

I must warn people, however: psychedelics like LSD *can* change one's personality. In some studies, researchers found subjects were more open, empathetic, and patient even more than a full year after their LSD use. The thing about being human is that change is inevitable. The only question is whether it happens in the direction that you choose.

 # Rachel's Words

I'm 31 years old. I do not have an autism diagnosis. Though I've always known I've been a little different. As a kid, I played with myself, had an active imagination, and lived a lot inside my mind. I grew up in a house where I was expected to follow the rules and get good grades in school. I always did my best, but often felt like I fell short of the expectations of the world around me. I just didn't get "it", whatever "it" was. When I was 10, I lost my mother, and my whole world was shattered. After my mother's death, life was different - there was so much she did for me, so much she knew I needed that I never knew to ask for - she knew for me.

I grew up being what was called a "tomboy" — I loved things that were typically associated with those assigned male at birth - Batman, video games, wrestling, bugs. I loathed dresses and pink. It just never suited me. After my dad remarried, I was expected to be different. I could no longer wear the things that made me feel comfortable. I was told boys and girls could not be friends — some of my best friends were boys. I felt soothed in writing, reading, and playing video games. Living inside my mind has carried with me into adulthood. However, while living under my dad's roof - this world, too, was soon no longer allowed. I came home one day to all my notebooks stacked in the kitchen. My step parent had read them all. My parents sat me down for an interrogation - I don't remember the words said, but I still remember the feeling. I stopped writing while I lived there after that. I found other outlets - some healthy, some destructive. All of it was a form of self preservation - to fit into the standards but also to protect myself.

This wasn't the only incident but I wanted to keep this brief and digestible. My childhood was painful. I always did well in school because I knew that was my ticket out. In my first year of college, I tried LSD for the first time. I remember the experience vividly, the way the world felt, the way I saw the world - I remembered the parts of me I left behind to survive the experience in childhood. It was a feeling that was so familiar, like coming home.

That was over a decade ago…

Nowadays, I still have a hard time remembering to find the positive parts of life...

Perhaps I have a hard time remembering to find the positive because of the natural human inclination and bias towards seeing the negative. Maybe. But it could also be that I still have difficulties because I lived for so long in an environment that did not allow me to be me.

When I was growing up, I felt as though I was suffocating.

But taking LSD let me breathe again. And for that, I am forever grateful.

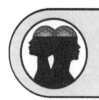 # Frank's Words

Microdosing ayahuasca was a desperate attempt to overcome the depression and loneliness that had enshrouded me since childhood. I had used psychedelics before, which opened up the world of spirituality to me, but the crushing depression and feelings of worthlessness always returned. I didn't expect microdosing to work for me, but I decided to try it and see what happened. Over the next few months, "microdosing" became "minidosing" — I would take just enough of my homemade brew to feel the effects, sometimes a little more, but always a small enough dose so that I could leave for work by 8am.

Gradually, subtly, my attitude towards life started changing — as well as my attitude towards myself. Maybe it was that one summer morning, with Bach's Second Brandenburg Concerto playing on the radio, when I realized it.

The ayahuasca had passed the peak, but I still felt this connection to what I had begun to think of as "divine energy." As the perfect harmonies of Bach surrounded me, I felt good — not just good, but exalted and transported. This moment, I realized, this moment in my body and mind, is purely mine. No one else will ever experience this moment — they all have their own moments, in their own bodies and minds. But this moment — and all the other moments of my life — were mine, and I was responsible for how I used them. I can sit here hating my life, feeling sorry for myself, or I can enjoy the pleasure of existing, of being alive and connected to the universe.
Just as the instruments playing the concerto harmonized with precision and grace, I was beginning to harmonize with the people and the world around me, after so many years of isolation. I felt I had received some secret knowledge — that life is magical, mysterious and wonderful. That judging myself for my social awkwardness was just cruel and unhelpful, and that I didn't need to do that anymore. And that nothing was really wrong with me. I can simply accept and love who I am.

Before my minidosing experiment, I had seen myself as a tragicomic character, decadent, broken, a failure. The best I could hope for was to find a conditional sort of happiness, having a little pleasure here or there, but not respecting myself or expecting anyone else to. But those mornings before the day began, listening to music, connected to the divine energy, changed everything.

I still have problems to solve, particularly insomnia. But thanks to the spirit-goddess of aya, I touched a deep source of forgotten love and emotion, and I learned that being autistic is not a curse. If I don't fit easily into the grand social drama of life the way others do, that's a blessing — because no matter where I am or what the situation is, as long as I can touch that divine love within, I will be fine, sporting a playful smile, looking forward to what comes next.

Juan's Words

My name is Juan. I'm 45. I'm Spanish. I was diagnosed with high IQ (132) when I was 12 and I found out (months later confirmed by a proper diagnosis by a specialist) that I was ADHD combined type. Lately, the combination of these two conditions is called "twice exceptional" or 2E.

All my life I felt (since I was really young) that there was something different about me. It was pretty noticeable both for me and for the rest of the world. I started speaking at a very early age and from the beginning I did it in a completely articulate, adult way.

The quest for discovering what made me feel so different has been something innate in me. Like an itch (as feeling different is not something you enjoy when you're 11), when I found out by the age of 15 that there were substances (LSD) that could grant access to areas of your mind that are otherwise hidden or unreachable during ordinary, everyday state of mind, I began reading as much as I could find on the subject. I was a "posh" teenager with no contact with any "dealer", so I had 4 entire years of theory learning before having access to the actual substance.

Finally, when I was 19, I got my first blotter and... it delivered. Not only did the LSD exceed all my already very high expectations, but it changed me for the better. LSD made me reconnect with a world that so far had made me feel like an alien. LSD obliterated any chance to lie to myself — as if it is a vaccine against self-deceiving; a great tool for a master-of-deception like my super fast mind. LSD also encouraged me to keep on digging deeper into my mind as all my previous efforts and hours of study paid off in a single night. I feel that being able to watch my mind and my experience from another point of view prevented me from the fate of other members of my family that became addicted to heroin, cocaine, alcohol, legal highs......

Psychedelics — as well as the strong science background and the level of English proficiency that my father forced me to acquire — have both given me a chance of being my own therapist. Even today it's very hard to find trained professionals in my local region to help with adult ADHD. And I know it's not ideal, but when there's no other option and your very survival depends on it... well... I feel this approach has worked well for me considering all of this.

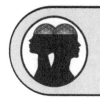

Belle's Words

Psychedelics awakened me to a life of possibility. I first experienced LSD in my early twenties, and the blinking stars in the sky invited me to zoom out and break free. After recently graduating from college, I had been described as "not a good fit" for my chosen career path (likely due to some obvious insecurities) and felt hopeless and stuck in a dysfunctional home.

Psychedelics led me to question old conditioning, revealed boxes I had been unconsciously staying in, and ultimately, introduced me to my true autistic self. I had been masking so well for years in attempts to blend in, but this contact with the magical allowed me to meet and embrace the mystical healer within myself.

My spirituality was awakened, and self-love was born. I soon traveled across the country in pursuit of my career dreams, and even earned several awards. While I may not have been a "good fit" in one professor's eyes, psychedelics helped me to gain the courage and confidence to truly shine. While this took repeated confrontations with personal/collective traumas and extensive processing to integrate, psychedelics' 'tough loving' presence helped make the journey more accessible. I am so grateful for my newer capacity to show up as my embodied, true autistic self.

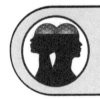 # Wanda's Words

My senses were overwhelmed, but I wasn't afraid. The reference points I had always taken for granted were being shuffled around. In the middle of chaos, I experienced myself for the first time, not as thoughts and sensations going through my mind and body, but as consciousness in which these felt safely contained.

I was aware of awareness. I was able to discern which aspects of my internal experience were intentional assertions of my will and which were passing scenery. Over a period of years practicing this discernment, I've become much less rigid and reactive. When I do react from a place of overwhelm, I am able to contextualize that reaction almost immediately. I return to a calm emotional baseline much faster. I understand what triggered the reaction. I know where I begin and end. I no longer spend hours a day ruminating or engaging in compulsive behaviors. As someone with autistic and obsessive-compulsive traits, this has been life-changing.

I notice intrusive thoughts. I feel overwhelming emotions. And I let them go. Sometimes I get caught up, but these moments pass. I do not identify with thoughts or emotions anymore. I identify with spaciousness. I am more comfortable in my body and with other people. Through these relationships, I have begun to feel more comfortable exploring sensation.

My world of possibilities has expanded, and it has not been a rootless optimism. It has not changed my desire for justice nor has it stopped me from fighting for myself and my community. It has left me with a new openness to having my worldview changed and a growing suspicion regarding worldviews in general. I feel a greater degree of agency to do something about the things I hope to change.

I have also become okay with decay. Accepting and embracing the difference between my strong ideals about the world and the complexity that is really there, I have become more attuned to subtler aspects of communication. I am conscious of my entanglement with my environment. I wake up grateful.

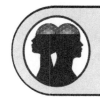

Victor's Words

Content Warnings: Discussion of Hallucinogen Persisting Perceptual Disorder (HPPD), Dosages / Dose Amounts Associated With Potential Adverse Response to Psychedelics

I was diagnosed with Asperger's as a teenager before it was reclassified under the umbrella term of ASD. Being more on the mild side, though, I felt at the time that it could be an inaccurate diagnosis, and didn't fully realize it was correct until later in adulthood. This meant I lived a long portion of my life with an affect deficit that I couldn't comprehend. Over time, I gradually began recognizing that others were attuned to a sense of empathy and interpersonal connection that I didn't possess myself — that is at least until it became painfully apparent that I was lacking something substantial; a fundamental component of the human experience. It precluded me from feeling a wide range of emotions, which in hindsight I would characterize figuratively as being akin to a robot or a machine, discerning and processing others' feelings within a purely logical and analytical framework, yet with no emotional substrate. At age 26, after reading about numerous studies on psychedelic compounds, I decided to try psilocybin and LSD. I used both on multiple occasions, and the effect they had on me was nothing short of life changing. They proved remarkably efficient in amending my psychological impairments and granting me that which ASD had deprived me of. I gained the ability to feel things which I very seldom had felt before, extending beyond the duration of the experiences themselves and manifesting as long-term changes to my emotional processing. I was suddenly able to truly sense love and affection, and also able to form genuine bonds with people and understand human interaction as a whole. Words hardly suffice to express the positive impact this awareness has had on my wellbeing.

Yet, along with these incredibly rewarding outcomes, I also got a touch of the more deleterious aspects of brash psychedelic use; a condition known as HPPD, which stands for hallucinogen persisting perceptual disorder. HPPD consists of semi-permanent changes — primarily of a visual nature but also concerning cognition and other forms of perception — reminiscent of the psychedelic state. These changes remain for a variable period of weeks to years subsequent to the acute action of the substance, in rare cases lasting a lifetime. This potential side effect ranges from mild to severe both in terms of intensity and in the degree to which it affects normal functioning. While some can easily shrug it off, others find it debilitating, and that is something that is not only worth noting, but imperative to spread awareness about.

In my personal experience following the overindulgent use of a couple of large doses of LSD within a short timeframe, I felt I was in a slight state of intoxication for several weeks. Not all of it was entirely negative; most effects I would label as neutral, if somewhat disconcerting, and a few were surprisingly pleasant — by which I don't mean to trivialize the considerable seriousness of the disorder, however. It progressively subsided to negligible levels over the course of months, with a few visual symptoms lasting years and still being subtly present to this day. While my case would be considered minor by most accounts, others suffer from this in a much more detrimental manner. For this reason, I believe advocating for the great amount of psychiatric potential psychedelics offer would be remiss without also speaking to the importance of responsible use. These are incredibly powerful substances that can make lasting changes to brain structure, and promoting their benefits should be done so in the same breath as furthering education about the dangers of their abuse. After all, such misuse is the principal notion that had them placed under Schedule I in the late 60's, unfortunately hindering scientific research for decades.

Psychedelics are neither inherently benign nor malignant, as many polarized views that prevail to this day may portend — rather, psychedelics are tools that must be employed with the necessary provisions and precautions to ensure a positive outcome. While everyone seems to have a different level of predisposition to encountering negatives such as HPPD, dose amount and frequency of use appear to be significant contributing factors. This is to say that more of a good thing is not necessarily better, and if someone is experiencing gratifying results from psychedelic use, the implication is not that increasing use will proportionally increase those benefits. Knowing when to stop is key. So also is spacing out doses in order to maximize benefits and minimize potential side effects. Most importantly, people should do adequate research before trying psychedelics for the first time. When utilized correctly, psychedelics can yield some of the most transformative moments of your life, which can lead to long-lasting positive changes that, in my opinion, may be unachievable by any other means.

AutisticPsychedelic.com

Qualitative Survey Responses

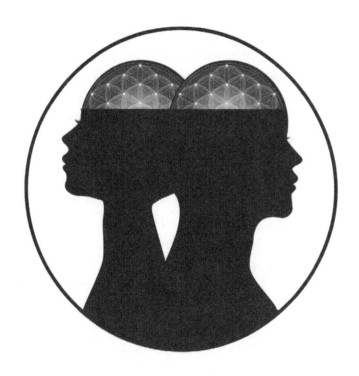

Collected Via

AutisticPsychedelic.com/surveys

Grace's Words

1. Bio (age, home country, diagnosis if applicable)

Grace. Age 30. France. Diagnosed with Asperger's Syndrome.

2. How did you feel / behave in the years before your psychedelic experiences (growing up, socially, etc)

Before my psychedelic experiences, it was very difficult for me to feel connected to people around me, as if there was a thin invisible wall between them and I, mostly because I had difficulties getting fully interested in their own interests and "reading their minds right". It seemed like I somehow missed some mysterious training in the interpretation of social cues, things that were unsaid but that you were expected to know. That resulted in plenty of awkward moments and resentment from friends or family, and I would not even get why they were annoyed or even angry — which of course made them even more annoyed. With time, I managed to create some sort of computing system inside my head, where I would visualise algorithms made out of memories of situations, discourse I've heard from people. This would work most of the time, but sometimes not — I guess because I would imagine everyone was thinking in the same way... ! Another difficult thing was sensory processing. I would easily get overwhelmed by stimuli around me, which could result in shutdowns or meltdowns. Overstimulation was generally provoked by these situations of misunderstandings between people and I. It was very frustrating for me to put so much energy into trying to "get it right" as it was laborious with little rewards.

3. Details of your meaningful experience(s)?

I had several experiences with psilocybin, san pedro and peyote. What they had in common is that they broke this invisible wall between people and me. During the experiences, I would be sharing a common perceptive experience, which seemed to be never the case before these experiences.

What was really stunning for me is that our perceptions would respond to each other, maybe through the power of suggestion. For instance, I would say "Wow do you feel that?" other people would respond "Yes," and we would just laugh and smile together.For once in my life I had the feeling that I was seeing the same things, understanding the same things as others at the same time they did, without almost any words, which was crazy for someone like me; someone who has had lots of difficulties finding her way through what's on the minds of others. For once, I did not have to laboriously create algorithms to understand what went through their minds, and all of it was happening on an intuitive level. Perhaps we were not having the same perceptions and thoughts, but it did not matter in the end; What counted was the feeling that "I was getting it."

During one psilocybin (truffles) experience and another one with peyote, what was really striking was the feeling of presence I held toward people and toward the surroundings. I felt a lot of joy, peace and life coming from all these beings, giving me a sense of unity with them. It felt as though, in the end, we are all made of the same stuff.

I remember being under a tree, and its branches were breathing and stretching out towards me as a friendly creature. During a peyote ceremony, sitting near the fire with other people, I experienced a feeling of presence that almost brought me to tears. These experiences were meaningful as they made me feel tangential to the world, in adequation with it, and not aside from it or outside of it as before. This filled me with calm and reassurance.

Another interesting memory during a san pedro ceremony: I was seeing small colourful skulls (a little bit like these colourful mexican skulls decorated for the Day Of The Dead) in each of the participants. Each participant had a skull of a similar shape, but with different colours, that I would correlate with feelings. That was another moment of experiencing this "Wow I'm getting it" feeling — no laborious computation, just immediate understanding. That was a relieving feeling.

4. Reaction / integration related to these meaningful psychedelic experience(s)?

I was afraid that these sensations of presence and "getting it" would fade the day after. Of course, all of my social interactions have not become miraculously great but it seems that I was left with some traces and memories of these perceptions and realizations. I still remember that the trees, the flowers, and the grass are breathing. I still remember this sense of connection between me and the beings, human and non-humans, that are all around me. I also know it is possible to feel as though I am a part of a community. I feel much less anxious in my social surroundings thanks to that feeling.

5. Feelings toward the psychedelic experience(s) over time?

These experiences have really had an impact on my way of being in the world and with people. Mostly, these experiences gave me a lot of peace in these interactions. And remembering these moments helps me feel grounded when I start to feel the first signs of impending meltdown or shutdown.

6. Notable challenges/difficulties of your experiences?

Sometimes I would worry that I would lose these sensations of connection and understanding of what everything "really is" whenever I would come back to what I felt was — during these experiences anyway — the normal "superficial plane of reality", a.k.a everyday life. I remember once telling myself, "Don't forget all of that when you come back to everyday life."

7. Perceived or lasting benefits of your psychedelic experiences?

As I said previously, I experience more calm and a sense of reassurance. I feel more acceptance toward my own limits as well.

8. In one sentence, how would you summarize what happened & why it is important?

I have made peace with the world in the sense that these experiences made me trust all of the world's components as well as my perceptions of them.

9. What's next for you in this exploration?

So far, my experiences have been really helpful. I've started to make connections between things and between people in a way that I did not manage to make before. Psychedelics also helped me to understand my own emotions better, which has not always been an easy task. This was mostly through microdosing psilocybin.

These microdoses would make me (1) have strong emotions, and (2) be able to analyze and formalize. Great news! So I feel it's a whole world ahead.

Hannah's Words

1. Bio (age, home country, diagnosis if applicable)

Hannah. Age 20. United States. Asperger's Syndrome.

2. How did you feel / behave in the years before your psychedelic experiences (growing up, socially, etc)

I didn't understand the reactions of others, they seemed completely random at times. I struggled a lot socially as a kid, conversations would move too fast for me and I'd be completely lost minutes into an interaction. When it came to my stimming for handling stress it became uncontrollable. I'd come home from school highly stressed and worried and to cope with my overwhelming feelings I'd go into a dark room and pace in circles for hours on end to relieve the stress I was feeling. My family was worried that I did this so much.

3. Details of your meaningful experience(s)?

On LSD, I was spending the time with a loved one who I trusted. The most incredible thing happened when I realized how much I felt for this person. I felt a strong connection to a human being for the first time ever and this caused me to react to this incredible amount of happiness (which I usually have trouble expressing) by sobbing from happiness for the first time in my life.

4. Reaction / integration related to these meaningful psychedelic experience(s)?

I feel like I can understand friendships fully and wholly now. Before this happening to me I felt like I was just just playing the part and not feeling much of the connection that I trusted was there. But it wasn't. After that experience I knew what I was missing.

5. Feelings toward the psychedelic experience(s) over time?

I cherish it so much and so deeply. I never knew how much I was missing until I learned that I, just like everyone else, need to feel a sense of connection that didn't seem to be accessible to me.

6. Notable challenges/difficulties of your experiences?

My anxiety still slowly creeps back up on me sometimes and I lose hope in myself due to my continuous struggle to find friends and friendships. I now know that it's not impossible for me but it's still hard to find connection.

7. Perceived or lasting benefits of your psychedelic experiences?

I definitely feel like I can notice and control my anxiety a bit more. The feelings of hopelessness in myself have gone and I'm able to allow myself to give it a try and reach out.

8. In one sentence, how would you summarize what happened & why it is important?

I finally saw the importance and raw emotion that can be experienced in feeling a connection to the people around me. This has shown me a new light in myself that fills me with hope and decreases my sense of fearfulness.

9. What's next for you in this exploration?

To address my anxiety — which comes back to me slowly and occasionally — I'd like to microdose along with going to therapy when I can to keep the strength to build on.

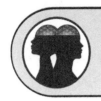

Nancy's Words

1. Bio (age, home country, diagnosis if applicable)

Nancy. Age 46. USA, Self-diagnosed ASD (have a child on the Spectrum & we are exactly alike). Clinical diagnosis: ADD, OCD, Generalized Anxiety Disorder, Major Depressive Disorder (MDD), Complex Post-Traumatic Stress Disorder (CPTSD).

2. How did you feel / behave in the years before your psychedelic experiences (growing up, socially, etc)

I was reactive, impulsive, much less self aware, less sure of myself and my emotional needs.

3. Details of your meaningful experience(s)?

Wow, hard one because they're so numerous.

Here is the most profound experience I've had while on mushrooms:

While tripping I looked at a picture of myself as a little girl. For the first time, I saw myself as that awkward, angry, sad. innocent, beautiful little girl and made the connection that she deserved love. I wanted to hug the young me in the picture. And, then I made the connection that *I* have to be the one to love myself as much as I'd want my parents to. Everything changed after that experience. I even had a desire to eat more healthful food!

4. Reaction / integration related to these meaningful psychedelic experience(s)?

Oh, these experiences have altered everything. I'm much more at ease sitting with discomfort. It's helped me with mindfulness tremendously.

5. Feelings toward the psychedelic experience(s) over time?

I need them less, but enjoy them especially if I feel I need a "reset".

6. Notable challenges/difficulties of your experiences?

Intense emotions, crying that I thought wouldn't stop (but it did, and I felt amazing after).

7. Perceived or lasting benefits of your psychedelic experiences?

Better overall mood, better focus, less anxiety, it's helping me deal with my fear of death.

8. In one sentence, how would you summarize what happened & why it is important?

Psilocybin is as close to a real cure for my anxiety and depression as I believe we will get.

9. What's next for you in this exploration?

More tripping when the time is right. Set and setting in 2020 = not optimal

 # Cynthia's Words

Content Warnings: Discussion of Suicidal Ideation, Condition / Symptoms Associated With Potential Adverse Response to Psychedelics, Condition / Symptoms Associated With Potential Adverse Response to Psychedelics: Borderline Personality Disorder, Mania Symptoms

1. Bio (home country, diagnosis if applicable)

Cynthia. Age 24. USA. Diagnosed ASD, BPD, & Gender Dysphoria.

2. How did you feel / behave in the years before your psychedelic experiences (growing up, socially, etc)

For a variety of reasons, mostly a lack of self-awareness and diagnosis, I was antisocial, depressed, and suicidal. I have never been close to my family, still am not, and I was also very emotionally closed off and resistant to beliefs. I was an undiagnosed kid who most likely was tested in secret by my mother at a number of specialists who hid the test results. I have since learned that I was just really good at masking, and that kept me out of finding aid. Couple this with a looming diagnosis of borderline personality disorder and discovering I was actually trans, and you could easily say my life has been constant turmoil and stress until I found LSD.

3. Details of your meaningful experience(s)?

I have taken macrodoses of acid, nearly every two weeks, for more than two years. My first few trips were not as introspective or illuminating, but it helped me understand my new norm of dealing with a high mind. LSD gave me the language, and desire, to start discussing the deep-rooted resentment and issues that had grown inside of me for so long, and it allowed me to look in the mirror and start asking the right questions. I've had a few bad trips & ego death experiences in more than two years of tripping, but I would have to say my most memorable experiences with LSD were the first time I accepted I was borderline, the first time I accepted I was trans, and the first time I accepted I was autistic — these were three separate trips at different stages of my personal experience, but each has kept me searching for answers to the questions I've had and been asking for years.

4. Reaction/integration related to these meaningful psychedelic experience(s)?

I had taken LSD a few times recreationally before actually entering into traditional talk therapy for an undiagnosed mood & personality disorder before I gave the diagnosis any credit. Prior, I was diagnosed with major depressive disorder with manic tendencies by my primary care physician. But within a matter of months, I was diagnosed with borderline personality disorder. Many of my earliest therapeutic trips were discussing and dealing with this new reality and recognizing the years of signs I simply ignored. This set of trips helped me recognize other areas of my life I was ignoring, and helped me understand that I am in fact trans. Another year of trips helped me grapple with that to the point I'm okay with both of these parts of my new reality. Once I moved away from my home state of Texas, I began to notice my reality unraveling at the edges while on LSD and started reading more about autism & getting involved with disability advocates and organizations on twitter. Unfortunately I have not been able to get an official diagnosis for ASD or anything near it as it will wreck my chances of immigration (as I am in the process of leaving the US), and having an official diagnosis will bar me from many things that unfortunately I cannot go without. I do not have the money for the testing either, nor even the desire for a professional diagnosis. I am a self-diagnosed Autistic.

5. Feelings toward the psychedelic experience(s) over time?

With my first four or so trips, I had not been aware that I could use LSD for more therapeutic goals, and instead was doing so recreationally as a risk-taking behavior, not knowing the long-term side effects. By the first dozen trips, I was in therapy, with my therapist's knowledge and awareness, actively using LSD in conjunction with traditional talk therapy. I met a few new people and we tripped together off and on for more than a year and a half with more intention than "having a good trip." I have had moments in which I've questioned the sanity of constantly and violently upending my mental state and psyche, but I've generally returned to the conclusion that my work with LSD is what is keeping me going. I hope to eventually do something with my own therapy & write about it to help others recognize the therapeutic effects of it, but really don't know where to go with it.

6. Notable challenges/difficulties of your experiences?

Entering any new therapist's office, I'm always cautious about the things I'm able to discuss there, particularly the fact that I'm a borderline (a "notoriously difficult" subject to work with; trans; and autistic), but I have been lucky to have accepting and supportive therapists in all three regards. Accepting myself has definitely been the hardest part for me, and linking my experiences with LSD to any of the "core tenants" of my life in fear of people no longer believing or supporting me.

7. Perceived or lasting benefits of your psychedelic experiences?

I am worried about the side effects and risks of long-term usage of LSD, and believe I have avoided many of them thus far. Even so, I feel that something as potentially volatile as frequent LSD macrodosing — which can sometimes seem a bit like the mental equivalent of sticking a fork in a light socket — could easily go wrong eventually. That said, I seem to have been lucky enough thus far.

I love myself and everything about me now — which is a major change from when I first began my trips. That said, I do seem to still experience a constant battle to love and accept myself in a world which clearly doesn't seem to readily or easily accept me.

8. In one sentence, how would you summarize what happened & why it is important?

I did LSD the first time because I was suicidal and wanted an excuse to kill myself, but LSD doesn't make you want to kill yourself — it invites you to stay and look around at the life you could have if you were happy. I'm not good at one-lines about myself or experiences, I think.

9. What's next for you in this exploration?

More trips, more writing, and more revelations about myself, hopefully.

Phillip's Words

Content Warnings:
Dosages / Dose Amounts Associated With Potential Adverse Response to Psychedelics

1. Bio (name, age, home country, diagnosis if applicable)

Phillip. Age 56. England. Diagnosed Autistic with ADHD comorbidity

2. How did you feel / behave in the years before your psychedelic experiences (growing up, socially, etc)

Mine is perhaps an unusual story given that I got busted at 15 for manufacturing pharmaceuticals, initially amphetamine sulfate and then latterly involved with psilocybin, LSD, eventually leading to freebasing DMT with a few other bits and bobs along the way. I was born before Autism was invented so my childhood was spent school-refusing or truanting. I had a collection of special interests from astrophysics to herpetology to veterinary science to organic chemistry. Not going to school didn't affect my learning. I just didn't bother with the O'Levels etc. My parents found me problematic so I left and lived in a squat for about 6 months before getting a lab technicians job at a university.

3. Details of your meaningful experience(s)?

Like amphetamine to people with ADHD, psychedelics just made me feel "better" at above microdosing levels. At microdosing levels I feel more focused, calm with mood elevation (not euphoria). Psilocybin is particularly good for memory recall especially from the distant past. Normally there are big gaps in my memory where I've forgotten things — psilocybin makes it easier to find things. LSD macrodosing is spectacular — a joyful experience and one where I'm particularly good at thinking tasks such as playing chess or designing things that don't exist (I've created several businesses based on these ideas).

Perhaps one of the most meaningful experiences was a kind of ego death where I was in an infinite space and surrounded by very bright, white light where I was in the centre and unwrapping from the centre as if I was a kind of fountain where each layer revealed a different version or character of myself at which point I remember saying either outloud or in my mind, "How can I be this many people?"

On reflection, I took this as a profound insight that allowed me to recognise the characters I had created in order to fit into the world and have excelled in multiple careers — as an educator, music video director, hollywood feature film animator, disruptor of the music industry, performer, and author — to the extent that today if I explain this "Forrest Gump' like existence to someone who doesn't know me the chances are that they'll assume I'm making it up - as indeed you may be assuming while reading this right this moment.

Overall, my most profound experiences have been when freebasing DMT which is an immersive experience that has helped me to consider the nature of consciousness as well as how the universe is constructed, e.g quantum mechanics and string theory. I've also had some of the best times ever.

4. Reaction / integration related to these meaningful psychedelic experience(s)?

Extremely valuable and allowed me to embrace who I am and those around me. I would be less happy today if I had not had access to these materials. They made me realise the medications that doctors and psych's had prescribed before I was assessed as meeting the criteria for autism were incorrect and it was this that made me seek formal diagnosis.

5. Feelings toward the psychedelic experience(s) over time?

As above. I believe these are extremely valuable materials, perhaps not for everyone but certainly for some of those who are neurodivergent. These days I perhaps trip two or three times a year — that's enough. If I'm working on a project I may microdose

6. *Notable challenges/difficulties of your experiences?*

None that I am aware of

7. Perceived or lasting benefits of your psychedelic experiences?

As above (see 4 and 5)

8. *In one sentence, how would you summarize what happened & why it is important?*

I have learned more about myself and the world we live in.

9. *What's next for you in this exploration?*

Research perhaps.

Jessica's Words

Content Warnings: Discussion of Suicidal Ideation

1. Bio (name, age, home country, diagnosis if applicable)

Jessica. Age 24. Norway. Self-diagnosis: Autism. Clinical diagnosis: ADHD.

2. How did you feel / behave in the years before your psychedelic experiences (growing up, socially, etc)

Very expressive with parents and a few close others, severe social phobia elsewhere. Highly anxious, depressive and confused 24/7. Every interaction with other people was confusing and severely stressful.

I have described my experience of living as walking on a treadmill set to move at random speeds, with a bucket on my head, receiving inaudible orders, then getting tazered every time I fail to follow said orders… Expecting myself to manage this AND be happy, thinking everyone else was doing the same thing.

I was confused, suicidal and very ashamed.

(I came off as balanced and snobby being quiet and weird.)

3. Details of your meaningful experience(s)?

I ate mushrooms of the kind that grow in Norway.

I was alone in my room and didn't expect much.

Tried to notice any changes in thought, but wasn't sure.

Looked in the mirror to see my pupils dilated and was instantly «tripping» by the sight.

Got a feeling of being convinced of something, but could still observe this as a feeling. Coming from a state of confusion and doubting EVERYTHING in my experience, this was a wonderful calm feeling I was missing.

It also felt as if I was sharing a secret with everyone who'd ever tried it.
The trip had a lot of elements, some uncomfortable ones too — but I appreciated all of it at last.

Then…

A kind of deity filled the room through the corners, and it was powerful and neutral in its intentions. It was like getting my unconscious projected on the walls.

I told myself «remember- acceptance»

The deity responded by coming on stronger- I got scared and thought «No, it wasn't an invitation!»... and then I got the irony and that I was still trying to control it.

Then I thought: «I've practiced acceptance, but forgot about respect».

I let the deity fill the room and darken my sight while getting visuals like driving in a snowstorm at night — but the snow particles went infinitely faster.

That was peak — on the way down I had some boredom experiencing superslow time, some weird sights in the mirror (I look like a frog apparently) and by the end…

I felt like a baby waking in the morning, fascinated by my hands and heavenlike light coming through the window.

Shorter Version:

I had first time experiences being calm, safe and certain in my mind. I learned that I don't need to control my sensory experience in order to stay sane, which is quite the opposite of the approach I had used earlier in life.

4. Reaction / integration related to these meaningful psychedelic experience(s)?

Read about psychedelics for about 3 years prior to my experience.

Two years prior I had a rock bottom experience, 20 years old ready to end it.

Met a guy at a party and we bonded talking about psychedelics for 8 hours straight. It was my first time feeling a shared reality, and I fell in love for the first time.

This was before my trip, but falling in love was so intense for me that I could find many overlaps to the psychedelic experience. This was also my first experience of wanting skin contact, and I think this also plays a part.

The guy I fell in love with taught me how to identify the mushrooms, but we broke up because he was indifferent and tearing me down.

It's important because it's a big first step in my journey and has similar effects. I think loving touch and sleeping together changed my brain to feel people as «warm» and not just threatening noise.

Two years after I had done a lot of mental work to « understand » other people / social relationships. I felt ready when I ate the mushrooms.

5. Feelings toward the psychedelic experience(s) over time?

Eyecontact: from zero wanted to sometimes enjoying it.

Notably less confused, more secure in my existence.

Able to bond with people in a new way, without compromising my authenticity.

6. Notable challenges/difficulties of your experiences?

After the trip I felt calm as I was facing reality. I saw peoples eyes and was almost attracted to them. I was less anxious overall, and still to this day I am fascinated by colours. The experience made it easier/more possible to meditate, like I found the anchor in my safe to stay calm. I can experience my states without being the states. It's like I have better internal communication in my brain. A lot of illusions were ripped from my arms, and sometimes I wish I could keep some of these illusions, but not really. I haven't really felt I had a «life» until the last few years. I don't feel doomed when facing challenges — I have seen my patterns and I trust my brain.

I feel like I should have a second trip by now, but it feels about as tempting as doing the dishes — if you get what I mean.

7. Perceived or lasting benefits of your psychedelic experiences?

Accepting my self, detaching from judgement, and handling challenges.

Social feelings: from pure survival stress to calm enjoyment and feeling people as «warm».

Overall feeling good things and passionate, where my best experience in life used to be relief.

8. In one sentence, how would you summarize what happened & why it is important?

I was integrated with my self and it made life enjoyable.

9. What's next for you in this exploration?

I'm entering a new phase of life and learning and I'm open to exploring my experience.

Nicole's Words

1. Bio (name, age, home country, diagnosis if applicable)

Nicole. Age 48. United States. Diagnosed Attention Deficit Disorder. Undiagnosed Autism Spectrum Disorder.

2. How did you feel / behave in the years before your psychedelic experiences (growing up, socially, etc)

- Isolated even in a room full of people
- Lacking a connection to others
- Limited in my beliefs about God
- Unsatisfied

3. Details of your meaningful experience(s)?

Awareness of God's true creation and how there is no real separation between any living being with a special awareness of the active spiritual realm — the fact that every substance in earth has energy and breathes.

4. Reaction / integration related to these meaningful psychedelic experience(s)?

- A love for my creator that is undisputed
- A connection to all living things
- A deeper acceptance of others
- Passion for not being a drone human
- Wanting to be with others who are awake

5. Feelings toward the psychedelic experience(s) over time?

Without these experiences I would feel like there is a lack of understanding. I would feel like the experience on earth was flat or fake. I am truly grateful that my experience was early (age 15 to 22) and then not again until in my 40s. I felt like it gave me an advantage over those who didn't know the connection we have to God and each other

6. Notable challenges/difficulties of your experiences?

Taking too much as a teenager and being afraid to do it again not realizing I could microdose and not feel out of control but just enjoy it.

7. Perceived or lasting benefits of your psychedelic experiences?

Oneness with all while acknowledging God is the master of the universe and feeling like he let me take a peek into the spiritual realm just enough for me to understand it is there and to respect it and learn more about it.

8. In one sentence, how would you summarize what happened & why it is important?

Psychedelics allowed me to understand that our experience on Earth is just a fraction of what is going on in the world and to embrace it without fear while learning about acceptance and love as we make our way to become more connected to God.

9. What's next for you in this exploration?

Legalization.

Adrian's Words

Content Warning: Dose Amounts Associated With Potential Adverse Response to Psychedelics

1. Bio (name, age, home country, diagnosis if applicable)

Adrian. Age 25. United States. Autism Spectrum Disorder.

2. How did you feel / behave in the years before your psychedelic experiences (growing up, socially, etc)

Anti-social except for I'd almost always have a best friend I spent most of my time with. I would act out for attention. I'd be openly verbally hostile for no good reason except to antagonize.

With family I was very quiet; they almost never saw me act like myself. My parents divorced at a young age so that stuck with me as well.

I was faking happiness and was a little prick a lot of the time. I was lonely even with people around and wanted to just be normal. I had no diagnosis until around age 19.

3. Details of your meaningful experience(s)?

DMT...

The first time I took DMT I had some very deep realizations. I entered a void of infinite purple/black emptiness and was pulled to a place with incredibly large geometric temples and disembodied voices that welcomed me home in a swirl of welcome loving embrace.

The voices gave me general advice for living and injected me with love and told me to be good and to spread love to others among other positive affirmations.

Every time since I've encountered at least one entity: a cosmic jester who takes me to "love school" where I feel as though I'm alone in a vast black empty classroom where I allow positive ideas and feelings to enter my brain and become part of my being. I also smoked a very large DMT dose.

Normally my visuals vanish with my eyes open and only DMT really produces many visuals for me. I opened my eyes after smoking and felt someone yell "close your eyes" before I did.

After smoking the DMT, I saw what I remember as an orange/green smoke swirl almost like a portal in front of me. When I closed my eyes I was welcomed by what had to be dozens if not hundreds of entities. A couple told me I was in over my head and almost all the others were welcoming me finally home. I remember feeling trumpets playing.

After that three or so entities surrounded me in an embrace and controlled the rest of the trip feeding me energy and love like a cosmic baby and telling me to grow as a person before I came back. I have tripped twice since then after taking multi-year breaks from DMT. They welcomed me back again.

LSD...

My first time doing LSD was shortly after my first DMT experience. I was at a friend's house and during the experience I had ego death and had about 45 minutes of panicking and showering in the dark. During that I eventually was overwhelmed by a sense of peace and I came to terms with a lot of my troubling childhood memories. I became interested in philosophy and spirituality after that but remain agnostic still today.

Mescaline...

I believed I was a tiger for a short time. This was a few months after my DMT experience.

Those are the most memorable experiences.

4. Reaction / integration related to these meaningful psychedelic experience(s)?

I changed the way I treated others entirely. I was finally able to get a girlfriend and maintain a relationship. I've had four serious girlfriends and am living with my current one hoping to get married.

I feel as though I'm an infinitely more open and aware and critical thinking person now.

I love life now. I love everything and everyone. Even things I don't like.

5. Feelings toward the psychedelic experience(s) over time?

The best things I ever could have done. I feel as though I may be dead if I didn't have these experiences. I was depressed. Now I love every moment of existence. Even when I'm complaining I have a smile on my face. Psychedelics saved my life and they need to be decriminalized for the sake of all people suffering who could benefit from these beautiful substances.

6. Notable challenges/difficulties of your experiences?

On LSD I've had thought loops and experienced paranoia. Nothing too horrible but people should be able to trip safely with a sitter.

7. Perceived or lasting benefits of your psychedelic experiences?

Love emanates from my every action. I go out of my way to help others now. Rather than to antagonize and harm, I'm able to live normally with my girlfriend. I wouldn't have made these changes on my own. I was too selfish.

8. In one sentence, how would you summarize what happened & why it is important?

I was able to finally see beyond the reality we build for ourselves. I saw that love and compassion are the purest forms of existence and strive to experience then every chance I get. It's important because without this I'd still be a walking shell of a person living in misery.

9. What's next for you in this exploration?

I want to be a person who pushed the boundaries of human experience so that I may help others. Maybe I'll become a shaman.

Zach's Words

1. Bio (name, age, home country, diagnosis if applicable)

Zach. Age 39, USA. ASD, Bipolar II, CPTSD.

2. How did you feel / behave in the years before your psychedelic experiences (growing up, socially, etc)

I was a deeply traumatized "old soul" autistic raised in a queer home in the 80s during AIDS. A neighbor tried to commit suicide and killed my classmate in the process. I struggled to make friends and spent too much time on the early internet absorbing misogyny and homophobia. I hated myself and everyone else for a long time.

3. Details of your meaningful experience(s)?

I've had multiple positive and one negative experience.

Mushrooms being the least harmful to my personal CNS.

A breakup while on mushrooms being the worst experience.

4. Reaction / integration related to these meaningful psychedelic experience(s)?

I've had neutral, positive, and negative experiences on mushrooms, LSD, 2ci or 2C-B (I can't remember now), something called "Foxy", and DMT — mushrooms being the least physically harmful to my central nervous system.

5. Feelings toward the psychedelic experience(s) over time?

I am still interested in plant-based psychedelics, I am no longer interested in manufactured or experimental chemical psychedelics, personally. Any psychedelics can be extremely beneficial, they also make the mind quite vulnerable again and I do not believe enough users recognize or revere that risk.

6. Notable challenges/difficulties of your experiences?

Each has its own difficulties. For me, chemical trips don't come in a small enough dose.

I am sensitive to everything, so most "standard" doses of any substance, including caffeine, are far too much for me, the exception being Novocaine apparently.

The biggest challenge after the negative trip and a subsequent trip into homelessness — because narcissists can't support people when it doesn't look good for them — was finding any help that wasn't faith based, let alone autism-centered.

7. Perceived or lasting benefits of your psychedelic experiences?

I manage near lifelong suicidal ideation by periodically reconnecting to my childlike sense of wonder and resetting certain mental patterns with this kind of "forced meditation".

It's frustrating that I have to go through unsafe channels just to keep myself alive.

8. In one sentence, how would you summarize what happened & why it is important?

Most of my trips had a positive — sometimes life-saving — impact on my depression and anxiety.

9. What's next for you in this exploration?

More learning and harm reduction work.

I'm also deeply interested in helping to communicate to the community the neuroscience behind tripping and what happens to our visual processing during a trip. I've had to explain it to several friends just to relax them mid-trip and it's helpful in remaining grounded and not getting pulled toward spiritual beliefs toward which they otherwise wouldn't.

Sharon's Words

Content Warning: Discussion of Suicidal Ideation

1. Bio (name, age, home country, diagnosis if applicable)

Sharon. Age 20. Hungary. Autistic?
(I was originally diagnosed as asp**, but it's an ableist term)

2. How did you feel / behave in the years before your psychedelic experiences (growing up, socially, etc)

I was always the "black sheep" — I'm closed up and toxic, and haven't had a day I didn't want to die since I was 7. I've always been told I'm rude and nasty, while I was just honest, and never said anything with ill intentions. also I'm very queer, which was — nay, had to be suppressed to be "accepted". My struggle was never addressed, nor were my limits ever respected, nor were my needs satisfied because no one cared. I always felt like a burden, and have been told numerous times I am one. I'm labelled a bad person, or "without empathy" while I'm extremely empathetic — I just have to suppress it because else it hurts too much.

3. Details of your meaningful experience(s)?

My second time on Molly (MDMA) made me feel genuinely loved for the first time in my life.

4. Reaction / integration related to these meaningful psychedelic experience(s)?

I almost cried, but then the feeling went away and I still feel like I'm hated by everyone ever, or at best, tolerated.

5. Feelings toward the psychedelic experience(s) over time?

I want more. Being sober sucks.

6. Notable challenges/difficulties of your experiences?

The ending — I almost started to get used to the feeling when it all fell apart.

7. Perceived or lasting benefits of your psychedelic experiences?

I can tell anecdotes, have experiences, and teach others about both the safety and the benefits as well as the downsides of substances.

8. In one sentence, how would you summarize what happened & why it is important?

I need to experiment more — doing so might help break down mental barriers I otherwise couldn't.

9. What's next for you in this exploration?

Molly (MDMA) preferably and/or blotter (LSD). I really don't want to learn about myself, but I really want to go solve some issues so that I can be a more functional human.

AutisticPsychedelic.com

Noah's Words

1. Bio (name, age, home country, diagnosis if applicable)

Noah. Age 18. The Netherlands. Autistic.

2. How did you feel / behave in the years before your psychedelic experiences (growing up, socially, etc)

Because of growing up with autism and not being able to keep up with the rest of my age (mainly socially), I started isolating myself more and more and at about the age of 12, I had barely any friends at all. At school I usually got made fun of and my grades got really bad. Everyday, after coming home from school I would vent my frustration with 'society' towards my parents and sisters which caused a lot of bad fights to happen. I pretty much saw everyone as a possible threat though I still tried hard to improve, knowing something was wrong with myself. I had barely any 'social energy', very bad social skills (though my parents did raise me to always be polite/have manners; shaking hands, smiling when someone is nice, introducing myself etc.). My filter was also really bad. I always tended to focus on the small details of everything and was very quickly annoyed by loud sounds or rough surfaces. I eventually got in contact with MDMA (couple of experiences, nothing extreme) and this, in the long run, helped a lot with my anxiety and having a better overview on social situations. It showed me an alternative way of behaving socially. This took about 7 months post experience.

3. Details of your meaningful experience(s)?

I found out about LSD when I was younger. I instantly got very interested (almost obsessed) with the substance, hearing about other people, their trips, and things they got out of it. I started working on getting some real LSD myself and after a while I was finally ready for the trip... I took LSD together with a friend of mine and we went to the forest. When we were on our way biking there I suddenly stopped abruptly and looked straight into his

117

eyes. I said "Man, you are god" and he, still on his come-up, was very confused. Then, after 30 seconds of the whole universe unraveling in front of my eyes, we decided to continue cycling.

We arrived at a spot but my companion wasn't very comfortable and said he really wanted to leave, so we left. When we arrived at my house my friend decided to check out some visuals that I set up beforehand.

As I was watching the visuals come to life even more I layed down on my bed and experienced (for what I still think it was) an ego death. My memories of that moment of the trip are very vague so I can't tell you much about it. My friend suggested we call another friend to hang out and we left my house. At a certain moment we sat down on a bench together and the village looked very peaceful, as if I was looking at a portrait. It all really felt as if we were in a dream. The friend that was with us (who was also supposed to be our tripsitter) took some LSD as well and we went back to the forest again. When we sat down at the same spot I decided to put on some Pink Floyd and go for a walk. I remember seeing the trees dancing around me and hearing the music not come from my phone but literally the sky, quoting: 'heaven'

I took another dose of LSD when we returned to the forest because I was already peaking and thought I could handle it and doing so seemed to mainly increase the visual aspects of the trip. After some hours the tripsitter guy left and it was slowly getting dark. I remember (trying to) explain some philosophical realizations I got during my trip but it was very very hard to find the right words. We both decided to go home and I had a very peaceful night of sleep afterwards.

4. Reaction / integration related to these meaningful psychedelic experience(s)?

I usually take a lot of time on my own and try to form new habits (or lay old ones down) but after my most recent LSD trip it was way, way easier to stop smoking and I realized that smoking was just pretty pointless. The LSD experience made me realize I do care about what smoking does to my body though before it didn't really matter to me.

5. Feelings toward the psychedelic experience(s) over time?

All greatly beneficial in their own way. Planning on having a lot more in the future.

6. Notable challenges/difficulties of your experiences?

When I'm with other people it still feels like there are still too many social rules and boundaries I must follow. As such, it seems I can't completely observe the psychedelic experience and be fully myself at the same time.

7. Perceived or lasting benefits of your psychedelic experiences?

Being more in tune with my emotions/able to control them much better. Feeling more connected to other people and therefore less isolated. Being able to look through people and detect their intentions significantly better. No abnormal irritation/feeling uneasy from external inputs such as loud sounds/rough surfaces/big crowds. More attracted towards nature and really being able to admire all the different elements of it. Different ways of listening to music; able to hear different layers in the songs and much more impacted by the emotion of it. More insight of what impact certain things have on me e.g. music, television, news etc. Calmer, more observing. I seem better able to — but also still sometimes struggle to — see the big picture instead of obsessing over details.

8. In one sentence, how would you summarize what happened & why it is important?

I have a better overall understanding and I'm able to see the beauty in life.

9. What's next for you in this exploration?

DMT. I've tried it once but somehow I'm getting pulled towards it again. I just really wanna keep bettering myself and psychedelics are one of the main reasons I can go through that progress with such a sense of flexibility. Psychedelics seem to make it easier to adapt to these new ways of thinking and taking on these new mindsets about things.

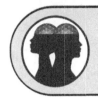

Eric's Words

Content Warning: Discussion of Suicidal Ideation

1. Bio (name, age, home country, diagnosis if applicable)

Eric. Age 24. United States. My therapist and I are both confident I'm an aspie, but I'm just now looking into getting a diagnosis.

2. How did you feel / behave in the years before your psychedelic experiences (growing up, socially, etc)

Big question. I think from the outside I mostly just seemed shy. I stared at my feet a lot and didn't talk any more than I had to. The most disruptive symptom to my life has been daydreaming. I create fantastical worlds or perfect lives for myself inside my head. Some form of stimming always accompanies the daydreams. Usually, this stimming would involve pacing and flicking my fingers. It would sometimes be so physically intense that my hands ached constantly but it was so immersive and pleasurable that I couldn't stop to feed myself, groom myself, or complete homework. My memories of life before psychedelics are a chaotic mishmash of daydreams and the nightmare of having to interact with the real world.

3. Details of your meaningful experience(s)?

My first experience with psychedelics was with LSD when I was 19. I didn't know I had Asperger's. My friend (who I now believe is also on the spectrum) was my tripsitter. The most notable revelation was realizing how powerful my mindstate was. My beliefs and perceptions completely altered the world around me. It gave me a sense of agency over my own mind. I realized how narrow and rigid my beliefs about myself and my life had been. I realized how my impulses and intuitions had dominated my behavior. I was able to "zoom out" from the nightmares and daydreams and see larger patterns. I understood myself on a whole new level.

4. Reaction / integration related to these meaningful psychedelic experience(s)?

There is an experience that NTs (neurotypicals) and NDs (neurodivergents) both have with psychedelics. Pseudo-intellectual platitudes all of a sudden take on new, profound meaning. For me, this took the form of my childhood therapist's advice. She would say things like "What if you look at that a different way?" but her words always fell on deaf ears. I would think "Who cares how I look at something? Reality will be what it will be." But all of a sudden advice like this seemed to hit home after psychedelics. I could connect it deeply to my own life. Selective serotonin reuptake inhibitors (SSRIs) and meditation both seemed to also give this effect a boost over time.

5. Feelings toward the psychedelic experience(s) over time?

I have only come to appreciate that first experience more with time. I am now convinced that it was not drug-induced euphoria because there have been lasting behavior changes. I am nicer to the people in my life. I work through pain and difficulty better because I am able to take the long view of a situation. After becoming interested in philosophy and spirituality, I have also come to believe that my experience was a somewhat mystical one with similarities to mystical experiences throughout history, drug-induced and otherwise.

6. Notable challenges/difficulties of your experiences?

My first experience was remarkably free of challenging thoughts. I had a very good tripsitter. At one point I responded quickly to something he said without thinking too much. I then realized that what I said had sounded harsh, and I then began to worry about how to correct it. I was paralyzed for a moment, unsure of what to do. My sitter recognized this and changed the music to pull my attention away from the discomfort. It worked and by the end of the trip I barely remembered this moment of difficult worry.

7. Perceived or lasting benefits of your psychedelic experiences?

About a year after my first experience, I had my first big depression meltdown in a while. I seriously contemplated suicide, as I had done often since middle school when I had attempted it. But this time I was surprised to find that there was a floor to my despair. A point past which I could go no lower. I felt that even if the rest of my life were pure misery, I still wanted to be here. Being here at all was a miracle.

I recognized these thoughts as being directly connected to my psychedelic experience. It is now four years since then, and I've never come close to seriously contemplating suicide throughout these years. This is by far the longest I've gone without those thoughts, and I credit that to LSD.

8. In one sentence, how would you summarize & why it's important?

I experienced the true meaning of seeing life from different perspectives, and it gave me an unshakable core of hope and love.

9. What's next for you in this exploration?

Since my first experience, I've had several others of similar magnitude. I've also tried microdosing a few times. I'm an analytical person, and I've love to find a concrete regimen to help maximize the benefits. I feel like society discovering electricity. I can tell this new thing is powerful and useful. I'm just not quite sure how to harness it properly yet. I've also been reading a lot of spiritual literature in the last year or so. It's helped me put into context some of the feelings I have that sound a little hokey ("the universe is love" "love and truth are one", things like that). I hope to keep reading people's perspectives on these issues and grow in that direction. If society can't accept "hippie" maybe it can accept "spiritual."

Walter's Words

1. Bio (name, age, home country, diagnosis if applicable)

Walter. Age 41, USA, ASD/ADHD

2. How did you feel / behave in the years before your psychedelic experiences (growing up, socially, etc)

I had no relationship with my own emotions. If anything, they varied from apathetic to pleasantly neutral. I was fairly disconnected from my family, keeping all communication fairly basic & superficial — unable to communicate what was going on inside. I had been involved with theatre since Junior High, which helped socially, although again, much of my connection with folks remained on a superficial level. By my late twenties, I started seeing a therapist because I didn't understand romance/dating.

3. Details of your meaningful experience(s)?

My first truly profound/meaningful experience was with ayahuasca at the age of 32. Words can't really explain the actual trip — again, it was profound. I didn't think humans could actually have that experience. The next day, I remember walking around feeling 'happy', It was a mindf**k — I didn't know people walked around just feeling happy for no reason. My relationship with my own emotions had been rewired. I felt I had access to ones that were blocked before. I was never much of a cryer. The afternoon after my trip, I cried from being overwhelmed by emotions — not in a sad, tragic way either. I cried the next day, too. Even 8 years later, it's not hard for me to cry.

The next night after my trip, I went out to a club — I was never one for clubs, but I was on vacation, and felt that's what you do on a Saturday night on vacation. I remember walking in, and just absorbing the environment in a way that was brand new to me. I didn't drink that night. Typically, I just would've gotten drunk.

I didn't go into my trip wanting to stop drinking. But my desire to drink was gone — and it was years later that I connected it all. I was drinking to dull the sensory overload I would endure at bars and clubs. I stopped drinking that weekend — I also stopped going to bars and clubs.

4. Reaction / integration related to these meaningful psychedelic experience(s)?

My ayahuasca trip started the journey that resulted in my ASD diagnosis (with a lot of mushrooms on the way). Psychedelics provided me with a sense of self and connection that aided in my introspective journey. Psychedelics helped me creatively. They helped me in therapy. They helped me listen to my body. They fueled in me a hyperempathy that I'm still unpacking. I walk into a room and I take in so much information, from microexpressions and body language to verbal intonation. I'm constantly decoding my interactions with people. Although overwhelming at times, this has helped me form more authentic relationships with a select few.

5. Feelings toward the psychedelic experience(s) over time?

I just don't know where I would be personally without psychedelics. They kickstarted a journey in me. As someone who masks with great ease, I never let anyone in — and I wouldn't give people any reason to think that there was anything behind my facade. Alone, it would be a different story. I would struggle in isolation. Psychedelics let me see how beautiful my brain was and appreciate the positive aspects of how it works.

6. Notable challenges/difficulties of your experiences?

Over the course of 20 years, I have done ayahuasca once and mushrooms approximately 15 times. I am lucky to report no challenging experiences beyond a bit of nausea.

7. Perceived or lasting benefits of your psychedelic experiences?

As someone who has struggled with alexithymia my whole life, psychedelics have really helped me build a better relationship with my own emotions. I may not always have direct access to them, but my understanding of my emotions is at a place where I can more easily understand them.

8. In one sentence, how would you summarize & why it's important?

Mushrooms and ayahuasca have allowed me to share myself with others.

9. What's next for you in this exploration?

I'm curious to explore other psychedelics, ideally with other autistics.

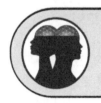 # Jason's Words

1. Bio (age, home country, diagnosis if applicable)

Jason. Age 25, Canada, OCD. Pursuing ASD assessment.

2. How did you feel / behave in the years before your psychedelic experiences (growing up, socially, etc)

I was diagnosed with OCD at a young age but this never sat quite right with me (today I am pursuing an assessment for Autism). I often felt this diagnosis was used to invalidate a lot of my overwhelming experiences that had simple fixes (like making sure my socks don't fold under my feet when I put my shoes on). I spent a lot of time angry around others, and sought refuge whenever I could in video games, a world I could control. As life's demands increased in my adolescence, I learned to suppress my needs and eventually started using cannabis to cope with the overwhelming demands of everyday life. I also started doing psychedelics at around the same time. My first time was probably around 15 or 16 years old, so my intentions with them then were not what they are now.

3. Details of your meaningful experience(s)?

Some of my most meaningful experiences were also some of my most challenging. Probably the most meaningful experience I've had was when I was around 19 years old. It was not in my ideal set and setting when it kicked in (at a University party on a busy beach a few months after ending a relationship). The psychedelics increased the overwhelming feelings brought on by my environment, which led me to seek refuge in a room at a house we were renting along the beach. The sounds of people socializing and having a good time below me had me confused about what I was even doing there. I had realized that I was trying too hard to fit in with everyone else that I was losing touch of who I was. The trip took a dark turn and I felt very isolated, alone, and misunderstood.

I started thinking about every injustice in the world and felt powerless over it all. Amidst this wave of darker thinking, I specifically remember connecting to a baby elephant whose mother was killed by poachers as the baby elephant was left grieving alone. I truly believed that I was feeling this animal's pain. As dark and gruesome as this experience sounds, the deep empathy I felt for the elephant that day made me feel more connected to myself and others. I realised that I didn't want to fake life anymore, and that I wanted to make real connections in which I didn't have to pretend.

4. Reaction / integration related to these meaningful psychedelic experience(s)?

I took this experience and allowed it to fuel my desire to enter the helping field. I became fascinated by the profound states psychedelic experiences are capable of producing and spent/continue to spend hours studying everything there is to know about them. Today I work in the field of harm reduction and am studying to become a psychedelic assisted therapist. I want others to have the opportunity to safely tap into all that these tools have to offer.

5. Feelings toward the psychedelic experience(s) over time?

Without some of my psychedelic experiences I wouldn't be where I am today. I often get trapped in rigid thinking patterns that get completely obliterated on my journeys. I feel like I am looking at the world with fresh eyes again. I find it most helpful to revisit past experiences in order to help reconnect myself to the lessons I've learned. I continue to carry these experiences in my heart with me.

6. Notable challenges/difficulties of your experiences?

I think the most challenging part of my experiences has been learning the right set, setting, and dosing for me. It took years of trial and error to figure that out for myself. I also think being on the spectrum increases the importance of set and setting for me.

7. Perceived or lasting benefits of your psychedelic experiences?

Over the years, I have been learning to accept myself for all that I am, as a queer neurodivergent person. I am learning to make meaningful connections and to bring these colorful parts of myself into all that I do. I honestly don't think I would've gotten here without these experiences.

8. In one sentence, how would you summarize what happened & why it is important?

I am not sure how to summarize how or why psychedelics changed my life, but I truly believe they are responsible for my ability to cope in a neurotypical world.

9. What's next for you in this exploration?

What's next for me is to hopefully be able to pursue an official assessment and eventually use my lived experience to be able to offer psychedelic assisted and integration services for other queer neurodiverse people.

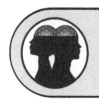

Diana's Words

1. Bio (name, age, home country, diagnosis if applicable)

Diana. I am 26 years old, from Argentina. I study Industrial Engineering. I do technical software and hardware service. I am autistic and I was diagnosed by professionals.

2. How did you feel / behave in the years before your psychedelic experiences (growing up, socially, etc)

The years before my first hallucinogenic experience coincided with my years without being diagnosed as autistic. I feel that I was 25 years working "in automatic." I really felt that I was a robot. I did not feel anything. I always thought it was like that and I was going to die without ever feeling anything. Also, most of the people in my circle considered me to be selfish; as if I only thought about me.

At the age of 24 I entered a depression or collapse, and before turning 26, I found information on the Internet about autism in women and I went with my mother and sister to an Asperger's association where they confirmed the diagnosis.

The first thing I felt was a relief because now I understood everything that was happening to me, but the following months I couldn't get out of that label and I thought I couldn't do a lot of things.

I recently began to go to the psychologist specializing in autism for children and adolescents, which helped me a lot and took me out of thinking "I am autistic and I cannot live in this society." Although, still, sometimes I continue having breakdowns and I have to use social masking to the point of overloading myself a lot.

3. Details of your meaningful experience(s)?

When I was 26, I decided to take a trip with LSD, at my house, with three friends, in a very careful and trustworthy space, after having read a lot on the Internet about LSD.

We took the LSD and our trip lasted 12 hours. The feeling I experienced was one of absolute peace, very introspective.

At one point I began to meditate and I felt a universal connection, as though there was energy flowing through many people who were meditating in the world at that time, and that this energy was passing through each one of us to be purified. It seemed as if we were cleansing the world of dark energies. And after that sensation, I began to analyze why the energy was going to be cleaning itself by passing through me — I asked myself "Who am I for that to happen?"

The days after the experience, I detected that what they call "ego shift" had happened to me, and that's how I interpreted it at that moment when I asked myself "Who am I to cleanse the energy of the world?"

4. Reaction / integration related to these meaningful psychedelic experience(s)?

In the weeks following the trip, I felt very calm with myself, and I kept receiving information about everything that had happened in my brain during that LSD experience. But I began to feel the big changes 3 months later, and I feel these changes are with me to this day, because I connected with meditation thanks to LSD. Now, I am meditating everyday, which allows me to live in the present and not in the future as I did my whole life previously. And all this makes my anxiety decrease a lot. I also stopped drawing conclusions about how others behave with me. I just live without drawing conclusions about everything — whereas before I was all the time over-analyzing small details.

5. Feelings toward the psychedelic experience(s) over time?

The experience also helped me to find again my topic of interest of all my life which is computing; to value the knowledge that I obtained in a self-taught way. The experience also taught me that I had quite denied myself the learning of certain subjects due to lack of self-esteem.

6. Notable challenges/difficulties of your experiences?

[no response]

7. Perceived or lasting benefits of your psychedelic experiences?

I would also like to say that I learned to say "no" to people when they need me — and this is important because this is the type of situation that I could not solve before; a common problem that generated a lot of anxiety and collapse for me. Today, however, I respect my time and my needs. This I think is a bit from the diagnosis and a bit from the LSD experience.

8. In one sentence, how would you summarize what happened & why it is important?

I feel like what happens is that I no longer have to go "plugging in" the part of my brain that I want to use, so to speak. Although I still have a hard time moving from one task to another, my brain is no longer so disconnected.

9. What's next for you in this exploration?

The next thing I want to do is a 30-day microdosing regimen. I still can't because in my country it is difficult to get pure LSD. I also plan in the long term to have an experience in a shamanic ritual.

Hope's Words

1. Bio (name, age, home country, diagnosis if applicable)

Hope. Age 42, USA, ADD/Depression/Non-Specific Anxiety Disorder.

2. How did you feel / behave in the years before your psychedelic experiences (growing up, socially, etc)

Highly introspective, socially awkward, difficulty reading social cues, difficulty understanding my own emotions & those of others. Empathy/hindsight/foresight were stunted.

3. Details of your meaningful experience(s)?

I've experienced several deep moments of ego-dissolution with the corollary being vast senses of interconnectedness, such states feeling way more real than ordinary reality. The dissolution of many internal walls in general has been monumentally cathartic with positive blossoming further corollaries.

4. Reaction / integration related to these meaningful psychedelic experience(s)?

These deep explorations into concepts of what I consider to be the true meaning, the core source of our consciousness revealed to be LOVE....well, this changes everything don't it! When one changes their perspective in relation to everything, then everything being perceived changes extraordinarily as well. This dynamic intersects everything.

5. Feelings toward the psychedelic experience(s) over time?

It's a category of experience for which I am deeply grateful on all levels. That such an experience is obtainable in the first place is just ****ing miraculous & that we GET to experience it blows my mind.

The part that I'm most thankful for though — the part that leaves me speechless, most often with tears streaming down my face as I consider it — is that we GET to share these experiences with each other. That we get to share these deep connections of love & healing with each other, creating waves of loving & positive momentum — THAT is the best part of the whole process!

6. Notable challenges/difficulties of your experiences?

Shadow work is always challenging, as it should be since it's the most rewarding. Staying focused within the psychedelic state is quite challenging but we have tools like meditation to help us tremendously in that regard.

7. Perceived or lasting benefits of your psychedelic experiences?

Deep Inner healing just changes absolutely everything that follows such healing. The benefits are infinitely all-encompassing whereas the detriments are vapidly minimal, at least in my experience.

8. In one sentence, how would you summarize what happened & why it is important?

Inner Healing births loving growth, and this growth births communal love.

9. What's next for you in this exploration?

To continue learning how to navigate peak entheogenic experiences. Besides the experiences themselves being incredibly rad, I am motivated by the opportunity to help others; to somehow positively impact others, and to birth love, empathy, and compassionate leadership into communities.

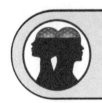

Charisma's Words

Content Warning: Condition Associated With Potential Adverse Response to Psychedelics: Bipolar Disorder

1. Bio (name, age, home country, diagnosis if applicable)

Charisma. Age 33, USA, no official diagnosis but have spoken with a therapist about suspected ADHD, Autism, and Bipolar II.

2. How did you feel / behave in the years before your psychedelic experiences (growing up, socially, etc)

Growing up was hard. I was an outcast and I never knew why. In late middle school and high school, I formed strong bonds with other outcasts who I now suspect were also neurodivergent. All of us had a strong sense of values, a distrust of authority, and difficulty fitting in. I experienced very strong, turbulent emotions.

During college, I got better at masking and figuring out how to fit into the world. I was still different, but I figured out how to make that difference generally pleasing to others — including those I worked with — and I also found ways to form communities in my personal life with people who were similarly different. Many of them were queer abuse survivors who were mentally ill. Took me a long time to realize how similar I was to them.

3. Details of your meaningful experience(s)?

In the summer of 2019, I visited a friend of mine who runs their own Psychedelic Experience business in Amsterdam who took me on as a client. I took an extraordinary dose of truffles for my first time and ended up with an out of this world experience where time stretched and nothing outside the walls of that apartment seemed real. I experienced my death and the death of the universe and saw the general shape of existence. I saw how small the issues were that I came in with questions about and left feeling a whole new sense of purpose in my life.

4. Reaction / integration related to these meaningful psychedelic experience(s)?

I spent the next year exploring my connection to psychedelic communities and spaces. I explored my relationship to gender, myself, and others. I wrote and talked about my experience with different people. I've continued doing smaller doses, working mainly with my nesting partner during integration.

5. Feelings toward the psychedelic experience(s) over time?

I'm very grateful for my psychedelic experience. I have experienced difficult things during and because of it, but I live a more authentic life now that I'm very happy with.

6. Notable challenges/difficulties of your experiences?

I definitely felt like I was dying during a part of the experience. I had read up on this and expected it, so it wasn't too hard to lean into, but that was somewhat frightening.

I didn't have a lot of nausea during my first experience but have had issues with nausea during some subsequent experiences.

One minor challenge was that whenever I was heavily under the influence of mushrooms, I was even less sure than normal as to what would be considered proper social etiquette. This caused me minor social anxiety in the latter half of trips.

7. Perceived or lasting benefits of your psychedelic experiences?

Extreme clarity in certain areas of my life. Creativity is easier now. An increased sense of connectedness with people, animals, and plants.

8. In one sentence, how would you summarize what happened & why it is important?

I went to Amsterdam and completely changed my perspective about existing, making it far easier to exist in an absurd and meaningless universe.

9. What's next for you in this exploration?

Gonna continue to participate in different psychedelic communities to see how things are shaping up over time as psychedelics hit the mainstream again. Keeping an eye out for ways to get involved that are both ethical in how I treat the world and how I treat myself. Supporting others who are interested in doing their own personal explorations.

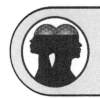

Cameron's Words

Content Warnings: Discussion of Abuse, Applied Behavior Analysis (ABA) Institutionalization, Self Harm, Suicide, Dosages / Dose Amounts Associated With Potential Adverse Response to Psychedelics, Symptom Associated With Potential Adverse Response to Psychedelics: Psychosis Symptoms

1. Bio (age, home country, diagnosis if applicable)

Cameron. 22. Nonbinary. USA. I was recognized autistic at 11 years old. I also have anxiety, PTSD, and depression with psychosis symptoms.

2. How did you feel / behave in the years before your psychedelic experiences (growing up, socially, etc)

I was a very anxious, semi-verbal child growing up. I excelled academically but struggled socially in school. I was relentlessly bullied, but often failed to recognize that I was being bullied, and then bullied more for being clueless.
I tried to kill myself for the first time the day before the first day of middle school, and had many more suicide attempts throughout my teen years, usually by intentional overdose. I had two TBIs (traumatic brain injuries) in middle school, the second of which also included a broken arm for which I received a hydrocodone prescription. I kept using painkillers after the prescription ran out because I like them more than my prescription for benzodiazepines (which I was prescribed for my anxiety).

Come high school, I went to an arts school for theatre. I like theatre because I was used to communicating with scripting already and have a knack for recitation. I was sexually preyed upon often, as I tended to make an easy target due to my naivete and perpetual confusion. I tried mushrooms for the first time my junior year, in the forest with two friends, and I remember wanting to write my college essays while on mushrooms because of how much clarity and optimism they seemed to give me. Then I tried MDMA at a concert, and it was the first time I had ever felt comfortable in a crowd.

One of my school accommodations was being released from class early so as not to have to navigate the crowded hallways, so this was a very big deal.

Nonetheless, afterwards my social suffering, painkiller use, and suicide attempts continued and I was eventually institutionalized for a year in an ABA facility. The treatment caused me to become deeply ashamed of all my past drug use, prioritized "behavioral health" over emotional wellbeing, and was traumatizing and isolating.

3. Details of your meaningful experience(s)?

Upon release from institutionalization, I went to a local engineering university. At first I was determined to not use any drugs, but this changed quickly when I was encouraged to try acid by a charismatic person who lived in the dorm below me. I enjoyed tripping because, in general, it wasn't any more overwhelming than everyday life, but everyone else would be super overwhelmed, so I felt for the first time to be the calmest one (and visuals are oh so lovely). However, one night this person convinced me to take an EXTREMELY large amount of LSD. I feel like being autistic — and also having undergone coercive behavioural therapies — definitely influenced how suggestible I could be throughout my life.

Even after that challenging megadose experience, I still stayed with this person for many more months. During this time, they often abused me and coerced me into taking higher doses than I was comfortable with taking. I melted down frequently, to which they responded with gaslighting and more abuse. The only reason I was able to leave that relationship was that my partner was eventually arrested and sent away to state-mandated treatment. I continued taking psychedelics on my own for a while after that, but about a month after my former partner was sent away, I vowed to stop doing drugs altogether.

4. Reaction / integration related to these meaningful psychedelic experience(s)?

After I was eventually able to escape that relationship, I started volunteering to help others through psychedelic harm reduction. For the first year or so of my involvement, I kept my pact with myself to not do drugs. However, eventually I started wondering if that was really the best option for me. I have since been able to reestablish my relationship with psychedelics and have tripped a few times, on my own or with trusted loved ones.

These days, I am very mindful about who I am around when under the influence. I much prefer small dose mushroom trips alone at home with my cats, making art and playing music and dancing. I am glad that I am doing psychedelics again. Mushrooms still give me the clarity and optimism they bestowed upon me that first glorious time in the forest. MDMA still helps me with crowds, and people in general, and I have been able to integrate such experiences into my day to day life and can channel the entheogenic feelings even when I am not on the drug. I have even done acid twice, both times with one other trusted person in nature. Both of those times definitely brought up the trauma I faced by being excessively dosed with the dangerous partner from my past; but they also made a deeper level of healing possible because being on acid again helped me reconcile with my own choices, and remind me that acid is not a monster, and that I am not a fool. The trauma I endured was not acid's fault, or my fault.

Many autistic people (including me) experience trauma, and many autistic people (including me) benefit from psychedelics, and many autistic people (including me) have had traumatic psychedelic experiences. All of these things can coexist.

5. Feelings toward the psychedelic experience(s) over time?

While institutionalized, I was taught to be ashamed of all parts of me that did not fit the perfect definition of a "healed" person, most centrally, to be ashamed of my drug use. This did a lot of harm in the long run.

Coercive, compliance-based therapies also influenced how easily harm could be done to me post-institutionalization.

This mindset of shame stayed with me for a long time, and I sometimes blamed myself for the abuse I faced because I was doing drugs at the time. This is a very harmful mindset and it is egregious and gross that professionals push it onto people.

Nowadays, I love my whole self, including my drug use. Drugs have helped me have a better relationship with the world around me - by helping me process anxieties, by supporting a joyful, growth-oriented, and optimistic worldview, and also by helping me explore my beautiful autistic psyche.

6. Notable challenges/difficulties of your experiences?

Psychedelic experiences still sometimes dredge up unresolved trauma, both from during my most abusive relationships and from traumas before. Drugs that have a harsher body load, such as 2-CB, sometimes send me into sensory overload on the come-up, and that can be difficult as well. In general, most of my psychedelic difficulties relate to bodily senses or trauma. While this is difficult, it is also important, and these days, the difficulties aren't dangers, only ways to unpack the dangerous situations I have been in before and bestow in me a deeper compassion for myself (who has been through a lot).

7. Perceived or lasting benefits of your psychedelic experiences?

I would not be me if I was not an autistic drug user. Psychedelics have helped me develop a deep and encompassing self love, accepting my identity as autistic and as a drug user. I adore listening to music and dancing with others while on psychedelics. I also really like playing with my comfort objects (both on and off psychedelics). Tools and toys I have long used for sensory regulation (like sand, putty, squishies, tangles, and other fidgets) become objects of intense fun and fixation for others on psychedelics, and I love witnessing the overlaps between autistic comfort and joy, and psychedelic euphoria. I have also found a wonderful autistic community, a psychedelic community, and an autistic psychedelic community that makes me feel seen, understood, and loved.

8. How would you summarize what happened & why it's important?

I cannot sum up my experience in a single sentence, and that is important because life is incredibly complex.

9. What's next for you in this exploration?

I will certainly do psychedelics again. The next trip on my schedule is for a solo home-based mushroom trip for Imbolc (a coming-of-springtime celebration), but if an opportunity arises before then, I might take it (depending on the specifics). Eventually, I would like to do an acid trip alone, and do a lot of journaling throughout the experience.

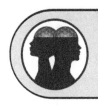

Maria's Words

1. Bio (age, home country, diagnosis if applicable)

Maria. Age 42. USA. Not asperger. I'm high-functioning autistic.

Did the 8-hour test.

2. How did you feel / behave in the years before your psychedelic experiences (growing up, socially, etc)

How did I feel? Like my whole life before doing psychedelics?

What kinda question is this? Xoxo

3. Details of your meaningful experience(s)?

I love God. She feels good in my body.

4. Reaction / integration related to these meaningful psychedelic experience(s)?

My whole life is an ongoing integration of all experiences of all kinds.

5. Feelings toward the psychedelic experience(s) over time?

Goodwill all around.

I love mushrooms, LSD, cannabis, and San Pedro.

They have been good to me every time.

6. Notable challenges/difficulties of your experiences?

Dang can't think of one negative, honestly.

7. Perceived or lasting benefits of your psychedelic experiences?

I'm still here and maybe I would've died from alcohol.

Psychedelics gave me a new lease on life.

8. In one sentence, how would you summarize what happened & why it is important?

What happened was I ate some mushrooms and god became vivid and I get to visit again anytime I want.

9. What's next for you in this exploration?

Tripping with friends when the pandem chills out.

Carla's Words

Content Warnings: Discussion of Suicide, Sexual & Domestic Abuse,
Symptom Associated With Potential Adverse Response to Psychedelics: Psychotic Symptoms

1. Bio (age, home country, diagnosis if applicable)

Carla. Age 48, Canada, Asperger's, ADHD, OCD

2. How did you feel / behave in the years before your psychedelic experiences (growing up, socially, etc)

I have Asperger's, ADHD, and OCD, all of which contribute to the treatment-resistant depression that has plagued me throughout most of my life. I was sexually and psychologically abused by my step-father and mother, both narcissists, and I am estranged from most of my immediate family. I first attempted suicide at age 12. I lived with almost daily suicidal impulses until about age 30. I had full-on psychotic episodes, oral hallucinations, and more — all of this while in my 20s and 30s. I drank alcohol daily just to be able to handle the stress of being around other people, though I never was an alcoholic per se. I couldn't hold down a job other than freelancing until about five years ago. I have not had an easy life.

3. Details of your meaningful experience(s)?

I have been working with a couple of different types of psychedelics which have contributed to a significant improvement in my mental health. I say significant but I feel like it's been nothing short of miraculous. I have experienced five large psilocybin mushroom doses, three LSD doses, and attended three ayahuasca ceremonies. I have also been smoking marijuana for several years, which has helped ease my anxiety considerably.

4. Reaction / integration related to these meaningful psychedelic experience(s)?

I feel neither a whit of exaggeration nor hyperbole when I state that psilocybin and ayahuasca have saved my life. I had tried various antidepressants and treatments over approximately 20 years, but nothing lifted my depression and improved my symptoms like psilocybin; and the few ayahuasca ceremonies that I have attended have also proved enormously helpful in being able to begin to lead a happy, much more fulfilling life. I feel like I'm living my life, as opposed to enduring it. My diet is much better and I exercise more. I can finally meditate and have been disciplined enough to do yoga. It all contributes to an upward spiral!!

It's easier to do things that I know are good for me. I'm learning to love myself and get rid of the shame that was embedded in my body for most of my life. I am simultaneously a different person, and more myself.

5. Feelings toward the psychedelic experience(s) over time?

I'm going to continue this line of treatment for another month, and then I'll likely take a break and attempt to write about it. I'm playing it by ear.

6. Notable challenges/difficulties of your experiences?

You have to be quite courageous to follow this line of treatment because it involves going very deeply into your own psyche. But the braver you are, the more you inevitably will benefit.

7. Perceived or lasting benefits of your psychedelic experiences?

I have been able to stop taking antidepressants and all medication. I am far more motivated and feel like I'm fully in control of my own life for the first time. I think the experiences helped to attenuate my ASD symptoms and develop socially to a far greater extent, and my ADHD symptoms have definitely improved as well. The OCD symptoms are proving more resistant, but are also becoming far less challenging day by day. I can plan for the future better, and have far better impulse control. The executive functioning of my brain has improved ten-fold. It's so much easier to live in this world. People don't confuse and mystify me as much, and I can understand myself and my own humanity far better than ever before.

8. In one sentence, how would you summarize what happened & why it is important?

Psychedelics have undoubtedly and greatly improved my mental health and should be the first line of treatment for certain disorders.

9. What's next for you in this exploration?

I feel a bit evangelical about psychedelics. I hope to help psychedelics become more socially acceptable, and hope to ensure that this latest development in mental health treatment becomes widely accessible to the people in my city who need it the most, i.e. those who are low-income and at risk. I have some attainable goals in this regard, and the ability to reach them. I feel like the world is my oyster!

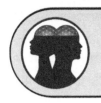 # Matthew's Words

1. Bio (age, home country, diagnosis if applicable)

Matthew. Age 30, USA, I am autistic, though I was misdiagnosed with a smattering of other disorders instead when I was young.

2. How did you feel / behave in the years before your psychedelic experiences (growing up, socially, etc)

I was socially anxious but outgoing around familiar people. It was not uncommon for me to put my foot in my mouth after having failed to read the room before speaking. I had to spend a lot of time learning to imitate the speech and behaviors of others to start getting along with more than my closest friends and some adults. My peers seemed to think of me as intelligent and trustworthy, but also dogmatic, and they weren't entirely wrong. Adults saw this behavior as ideal, and I only seemed to deviate from it occasionally, typically when I thought something was unjust or unfair. I would say it's fair to say I was rigid and calculating, but also warm in a stiff sort of way.

3. Details of your meaningful experience(s)?

During the first experience, I felt at peace in a way that I rarely have, if ever. I didn't feel at one with my body, but for the first time in a long time, maybe ever, I was not at odds with it — at least not in the usual way. I've felt trapped or cursed with a body that doesn't match me, so I've historically mistreated it. I hadn't made this type of realization in more than a passing, intellectual way prior to this. But during the experience, I was calm. And that's an exceedingly rare sensation for me.

My second meaningful experience could be categorized as a bad trip, but I benefited from it. I came to terms with my sexuality, I cried, and I came out to my parents as bisexual.

The term "bisexual" is not entirely accurate, but it is a term they could understand. I knew my mom would be supportive, but my dad is well known for being homophobic, so I was scared. I kept having this image flash through my mind of me introducing a boyfriend to him, imagining that my dad would then shoot this boyfriend. I kept thinking that I would rather he shoot me than refuse to love me for who I am. Then a thought came to me... "Kind people deserve the chance to be kind, and we deserve the chance to be disappointed by the unkind. You can't be disappointed by what you always expect." If I've ever heard the voice of God, it was in that moment. So I came out to my dad. He made an off color joke, double checked if I was serious, then told me he loved me. Always.

4. Reaction / integration related to these meaningful psychedelic experience(s)?

I am still anxious, frequently suffer depressive episodes, and am not great at reading the room. However, I am more able to live in my body than before. I feel that I have gained a kind of patience and wisdom that I didn't have before; a willingness to let things go, and the ability to do so — more than before, anyway. Also, I am more honest with myself, I think.

5. Feelings toward the psychedelic experience(s) over time?

I am thankful for these experiences.

I am a better person for having had them, even the difficult ones.

I would say that it is like experiencing 6 months of therapy in 8 hours. You're not skipping any of the difficult parts, just moving through them quickly.

6. Notable challenges/difficulties of your experiences?

Very few, if any.

The digestive distress is something but I didn't really care about that during the experience.

7. Perceived or lasting benefits of your psychedelic experiences?

I am more in tune with my body and more open to nature than I was previously. There is more of a sense of oneness with the universe rather than the sense of feeling entirely separated from it. It is difficult to hide from yourself during a psychedelic experience, and while confronting yourself can be difficult, it is worth doing.

8. In one sentence, how would you summarize what happened & why it is important?

I grew into a better version of myself, and that is something that we should always be working towards.

9. What's next for you in this exploration?

I don't know, and that's okay.

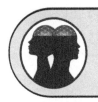

Don's Words

1. Bio (age, home country, diagnosis if applicable)

My name is Don. I am 43 years old, from England, and was diagnosed with Autism Spectrum Disorder and ADD, just one year ago.

2. How did you feel/behave in the years before your psychedelic experiences (growing up, socially, with family, etc)

I felt like an outsider, looking in — almost as though I spoke a different language to my neurotypical peers. I have always related to neurodiverse people better. I would often get irritable and frustrated with people and with life.

I think I have always been able to read body language and facial expressions, but have often been mystified as to why people think, feel or behave a certain way. I could see that someone was unhappy, or cold, with me, but, often, I did not know why.

I can sometimes be outspoken and unintentionally offend, or rub people up the wrong way. I have experienced a lot of difficulty controlling my emotions and this has impacted my relationships.

3. Details of your meaningful experience(s)?

I have had so many, over the years. I first began to use psychedelics as a teenager. However, we didn't know anything about set and setting and, although we had a lot of fun, we also had some negative experiences, bad trips, or became paranoid. I was later to abandon psychedelics, in lieu of drugs that just made me feel nice and did not involve any inner work. I eventually came full circle, rediscovering psychedelics, as an adult, after quitting the hard drugs and alcohol, I had been abusing — to mask my autistic symptoms.

Psychedelics and cannabis have made me more conscious of my defects and helped me to take a step back from myself – in order to react to situations in a calmer and more conscientious way. I have not used hard drugs or alcohol, in five years. My last meaningful experience was a macro dose of magic mushrooms. I feel like it positively reorganized my brain.

4. Reaction/integration related to these meaningful psychedelic experience(s)?

I have become more aware of myself and my behavior. I feel I am more empathetic. I find myself in confrontation a lot less often and my symptoms have lessened — in particular, I noticed I was stimming and scripting a lot less. This made me realize that these two symptoms, at least in my case, are caused by negative thought loops. Therefore — I am experiencing fewer invasive thoughts.

5. Feelings toward the psychedelic experience(s) over time?

I look back fondly on these experiences and also feel proud for having plucked up the courage to take some of the larger doses.

6. Notable challenges/difficulties of your experiences?

Sometimes, the chatter in my mind became a little irritating, but I got through it, by surrendering to the experience and meditating, on my breath, while enjoying the closed eye visuals.

7. Perceived or lasting Benefits of your psychedelic experiences?

The aftereffects, from my last experience, seem to be getting better, every day. I have had very few emotional outbursts and am more patient.

8. In one sentence, how would you summarize what happened & why it is important?

I feel as though I was rebooted – this is important to me, because I was tired of the old thought patterns and want to get on with people better.

9. What's next for you in this exploration?

I shall continue to use psychedelics, periodically. I find the positive effects can last a few weeks, until I feel I could benefit from another booster. There is so much more to explore.

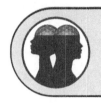

Stephen's Words

1. Bio (age, home country, diagnosis if applicable)

Stephen. Age 27, United States, Asperger's/Synesthesia

2. How did you feel / behave in the years before your psychedelic experiences (growing up, socially, etc)

I grew up sort of living two different types of lives as the result of a divorce between my parents. On one side I was living a sheltered life with little socialization and exploration, while on the other side I was encouraged to live more freely. I think I didn't know how to do the latter. There's a lot of mixed messages that come through when you're raised in a nuclear family environment, as I did when both of my parents remarried. I feel that I was overwhelmed at most points in my experience. I grew up very shy and had most things done for me so I was a late bloomer, too. Neither of my parents know I had autism (or synesthesia for that matter), even though I stimmed pretty openly. None of us understood what was going on with me. The nuclear environment likely contributed to my depression as I grew up. I'm also genetically predisposed to depression, but not being understood in my autism didn't make it any easier. I got on antidepressants around 20 years of age and I didn't like how they made me feel. I couldn't feel any "highs" or any "lows," either, but I could rage and I just wasn't happy. Communicating and connecting with others was already hard for me and the antidepressants made me feel like even more of a martyr. I gradually weaned myself off of the meds maybe a year later and started practicing Buddhism and mindfulness.

3. Details of your meaningful experience(s)?

Shortly after I weaned myself off the meds, I had the chance to experience LSD with a veteran psychonaut. We went out into nature at a local park by the water and proceeded into a journey that lasted about 6 or 7 hours.

I remember it as the best day of my life. I was nervous, going into it, about what I'd heard about hallucinations. I didn't want to have a bad trip, but my guide assured me the hallucinations weren't anything like I'd heard. And they weren't. I remember a sort of "shaking" feeling in my stomach coming on, feeling my head get lighter, and then finally looking at this little twig on a tree shaking in front of me, but in a different way than normal. I could feel the energy of this twig and it was a joyous little twig! So excited to be alive in nature! I started to connect with all sorts of nature surrounding me; the ferns and the trees. Even the spiders beneath the ferns.

I felt like we were all on a sort of grand adventure together and we were. I could see these thread-like connections all throughout the forest, connecting a leaf to another leaf or a fern. I could see all of these connections (and still do, thanks to my synesthesia). I stared out at the water at one point, which was the most beautiful blue I'd ever seen, and all of a sudden I got hit with this insight. All of my studies with Buddhism and the concept of Emptiness (or Sunyata) suddenly made sense. And I cried. It's one of my most cherished memories.

I had several psychedelic experiences after this, but the most important was when I sat with ayahuasca for the first time. In ayahuasca, I was able to really connect with my synesthesia and see these metaphorical blocks that it created for me as defense mechanisms, in cahoots with my autism. In particular, I discovered that I was living according to video game rules of communication. Sounds like a joke. Isn't a joke. Like many autistics, I used media to make sense of reality. The computer was my safe space as a kid and I played a lot of The Sims. I loved how I could make people get along with each other so easily in that game according to a "formula" using their methods of communication. My synesthesia took this template and tucked it into my subconscious for use. I didn't realize I was using a communications template from a video game for all those years until ayahuasca. It was wild. That was only a few years ago. I always knew something was "off" about my communication, but I didn't ever think it could be something like that.

4. Reaction / integration related to these meaningful psychedelic experience(s)?

That first experience with LSD was just a joy. I was so happy to know that all of the mystical beliefs I'd incorporated into my life weren't for naught. I certainly rode the high of that trip for many months after. However, I also kept "chasing the dragon" or looking for that same experience over and over again. I certainly had many blissful journeys afterward, but I think what I would say to my past self now is, "Take it slow! Let yourself integrate one experience fully before diving into another one. Also, not everyone is going to 'get it' when you talk to them about this stuff and that's okay. Everyone has their way and it doesn't have to match up with your own."

The ayahuasca journey was much harder to integrate. It was a very intense experience. There was a lot in that trip that was made clear and I realized that a lot of things in my life didn't add up to the life that I was feeling called to live. I became othered from my friend group, which was some of my own doing, because I realized we didn't fit so well together, anymore. I think the communication aspect of that journey has been a long one, though, still evolving to this day. I felt like I had to start over from scratch with how I related to people. My communication has improved greatly since, but it has become something I am highly aware of in myself and in others.

5. Feelings toward the psychedelic experience(s) over time?

I've always been fond of it. I tell people it feels like home to me. As a synesthete, my senses already cross like they do in the psychedelic realm, so it feels wonderful to be in a dimension where that is more "acceptable." I think that existence is inherently psychedelic, so I don't have to be in that realm to appreciate it as much, anymore. It's been great to have so many veils lifted over the years.

6. Notable challenges/difficulties of your experiences?

I'm a very anxious person. It's probably in my genes. Almost every single time I've been in the psychedelic space, I worry about my heart rate. I have to laugh though, because this is a very normal thing across the map. I've learned to just "breathe and trust" during those lapses of doubt. Most of the time that works, but I did have one experience where I spun way out and panicked. Thankfully I had a guide with me and just said, "I think I need some help," and they came and held me in their arms and rocked me like a baby and just fed me so much love. Even though it was a scary experience, it was one of the most essential I've had. It taught me just how strong the power of love is.

7. Perceived or lasting benefits of your psychedelic experiences?

So many! Better communication skills, increased awareness, increased focus, an acceptance and celebration of my autism and synesthesia, an enduring oneness mindset. I eat healthier. I love water. I have a sense of where my ground/my center is and have an easier time finding my way back to my "self" when I fall off the wagon. I treat myself with more gentleness. I practice magic very openly instead of being closeted.

8. In one sentence, how would you summarize what happened & why it is important?

I became integrated with Source, which is Love, and I learned that I am part of a VERY intricate web of interconnectedness where we're all just doing the best we can and we have to be easy on ourselves because let's be real; it's a lot and we're always looking out for ourselves, even our unconscious / subconscious tendencies.

9. What's next for you in this exploration?

I just started school, majoring in Psychology. The plan is to pursue a career as a psychedelic therapist later on down the road. But while that seed is being nurtured, I'm finishing up on my first book, which is about my psychedelic experiences and how they helped me. I am also trying to organize harm reduction/integration circles right now. Other than that, I am open to what the Universe has in store for me.

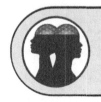

Elliot's Words

1. Bio (age, home country, diagnosis if applicable)

Elliot. Age 38. United States. Diagnosis: Asperger's or High-Functioning Autism Spectrum Disorder.

2. How did you feel / behave in the years before your psychedelic experiences (growing up, socially, etc)

Assuming the question is aiming to contrast specific qualities and behaviors pre- and post-psychedelic experience, I guess I'd have to say that I was primarily detached and cold in human relationships, feeling alien, ill-equipped for social dynamics, and physically and intellectually at odds — my mind and conscious disconnected and out of sync with my physical body. Being autistic is much like being left-handed in the right-handed world we have: you make millions of adjustments every day to fit in and hide all the unnatural, awkward tendencies of your biology, half of the time unaware that there could be a different way.

I was/am an alien among the humans, constantly honing my personas to blend in and stay out of detection, losing friends and lovers along the way who got too close and were burned by my inability to hold up my many facades. The feelings of alienness, the disconnection from my body — and inability to authentically connect with my persona or personality — led me to various states of mental instability and emotional constipation. My tendencies for extremism came out in philosophical, spiritual, and psychological research, as well as in sociology, anthropology, and urban/community planning as ways to understand humans more and keep convincing myself I had a place in the human drama.

3. Details of your meaningful experience(s)?

One of my earliest experiences introduced me to the concept of unconditional love, and the yogic paths of unity, and how all life is ritual to this end. I saw everything as a practice that we perpetuate our intentions with and create or manipulate as a god/creator does with infinite and wise energy. Yoga or Unity, whatever the path (bhakti, jnana, karmic, or raja etc) all require the same practice of pressing through. Just different methods of pressing into more unity.

In another experience, I understood Christ consciousness for the first time. I saw how Krishna and Christ are one, and as is said in various ways through Hinduism, Judaism, and Islam, god is one. I saw myself as god, too.

I understood that the universe is as one; all things reflections of these karmic desires for unity. This brought out new ways to look at relationships and have appreciation/love for others, forever changing my ideas about work, service, and art.

Another experience was having been visited/inhabited by sacred animal elders. The animals that visited me combined consciousnesses with me after I'd had a Kundalini experience and taught me many things about them and about myself. I connected to primal aspects of my self and my species, and felt more unified with the earth and all living things. I felt great healing and expanded openness to being a human. I understood presence for the first time and this has changed my life, as now I don't feel such a slave to space/time anymore. I feel more 'in my body.' The practice of presence, as cliche as it is, is the path to heaven, to happiness, or unity.

One of my last experiences taught me that all these psychedelic experiences are just experiences. They are wonderful experiences, but are like little previews for the grand event. They are temporal, are subject to space and time, and live only as a reminder to seek greater unity with god. Experiences for experience sake is dualistic because it puts me in a role as an experiencer and takes me out of the relationship of presence. This has instilled in me that daily practices and habits are the way to lasting wokeness, and to rely on my growing strength of character and spirit to navigate this world.

4. Reaction / integration related to these meaningful psychedelic experience(s)?

Many experiences have got me to reconnect with my physical body. People with ASD typically have trouble with this and I think this is part of the reason why we also get caught in the ever-solidifying realities we make up with our rich intellectual world. Because this alienates us further.

In learning to reconnect physically, I've learned to incorporate healthier environment conditions in my home/work, to incorporate more physical touch with family/friends, and to establish new and healthier practices with lovers. These awarenesses have also helped me develop more unique skills with my senses as a cook, a musician, and also as a visual artist.

Many of my opinions about humanity and my ability to be an authentic part of it were very bleak before. After some psychedelic experiences, I've been able to empathize more with humans and feel more comfortable being my awkward or quirky self. My growing confidence in how to appreciate, love, and support my self (in all my unique neurodiverse ways) has allowed me to better see different paths toward appreciating, loving, and supporting those around me.

I've integrated many daily practices like meditation, prayer, movement (dance/yoga), and music/voice over the years. These practices ground me and create stability of mind and spirit so driving or going to a grocery store can feel more manageable. When I feel my autistic freakouts starting to build (cuz I'm recognizing them in my body quicker/sooner), I can adapt with more patience and success.

5. Feelings toward the psychedelic experience(s) over time?

Like I mentioned above, I'm learning that psychedelic experiences are just experiences. They have a time/place, but they are a fine tool if used well, and a distraction if used unwell. I think natural psychotropics or entheogens are the best tools and should always be done with intention. Plants carry in them great wisdom and tradition and the further I progress with plant medicines, the more I am blown away with how interconnected and wise these teachers really are.

Communities for integration and support are essential and really should be promoted as the most important aspect of the psychedelic experience. I think plant-based psychedelics should be decriminalized and that indigenous traditions of plant use should be supported. I also think that clinical research for the further adoption and use of entheogens in medical practices should be sought with fervor. But I fear exploitation and power manipulation in any markets that grow out of these and ensuing political and cultural backlashes.

6. Notable challenges/difficulties of your experiences?

Not for me.

7. Perceived or lasting benefits of your psychedelic experiences?

I feel more connected with myself and others — as though I have a real foundational understanding of what that looks like, feels like, sounds like. I still struggle, but less so than I used to. And I always have this ground level I'm familiar with — a level to which I know I can return.

To feel disembodied your entire life and then finally experience it is unlike anything I've ever known. This awareness has allowed me to find meaning in this thing we call existence. Depression will still come and go, but it does not have the same weight it used to.

8. In one sentence, how would you summarize what happened & why it is important?

Psychedelics provided me experiences of what many call enlightenment, union, or christ consciousness, providing a lens by which to view a new reality that I didn't have words or a vision for previously, thus impacting me irreversibly into action for a more connected, deep, and vibrant relationship to life.

9. What's next for you in this exploration?

I'm looking to have another experience, but hopefully on my own terms, and in a positive environment.

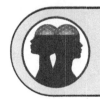

Pete's Words

Content Warnings: Discussion of Near-Death Experience,
Dosages / Dose Amounts Associated With Potential Adverse Response to Psychedelics

1. Bio (age, home country, diagnosis if applicable)

Pete. United States, ASD diagnosis but I identify as neurodivergent.

2. How did you feel / behave in the years before your psychedelic experiences (growing up, socially, etc)

I always felt like a black sheep. I had a pattern of making friends and then eventually having them "unfriend" me and I never understood why. My folks had my hearing tested when I was 5 because they were convinced something was wrong. It turned out I just was so hyper-focused on whatever I was doing that I would unintentionally tune them out. This tendency was misconstrued as being willfully rude and naughty and would get me punishments including spanking. I would get belted now and again when I would have meltdowns, like the time when my mom's cactus popped my basketball so I destroyed the cactus with a shovel that was nearby. I also had Tourrette's tics that would come out in jerky full body motions when I was especially anxious, so my parents would make sure that I always had something to occupy my hands (e.g. suspenders). I never knew why I was so averse to bright sunlight and loud sounds like sirens/alarms. My special interest until age 12 was basketball and I would sleep with my ball every night. I worshipped Pistol Pete Maravich and would practice his ball-handling drills and tricks until my hands would bleed. I have since come to realize that there was a good chance he was undiagnosed as being on the spectrum himself, which makes a lot of sense! I would listen to the same Elton John cassette on a loop for a few years between age 6 and 8.

In adolescence I was always way too socially anxious to ask girls out but in my senior year of highschool a girl asked me to a dance and we dated for a while. I developed pretty bad irritable bowel syndrome as a teen and was constantly stressed and worried about having an episode during times when there might not be a bathroom nearby.

I ruminated on this happening constantly and did have a few close calls with bathroom emergencies. No one thought I needed help with my anxiety like getting therapy at the time since this was stigmatized and meant there was something "wrong" with you.

I was obsessed with music and would insist on bringing my heavy books of hundreds of cds with me most places I went. This drove my parents crazy on vacations — as one might imagine! I really internalized mixed messages from my family and teachers that I was "gifted" and "special" but also that I lacked common sense and social skills. I found this incongruence very confusing and frustrating of course, and assumed there was just something wrong with me fundamentally. Despite graduating from my prestigious college prep school with a 3.8 GPA and getting accepted to several colleges including the prestigious Berklee College of Music, I was nonetheless chosen as "most likely to live with their parents in 10 years" by whoever organized the senior yearbook at my high school. This prediction ended up being quite prescient, sadly. Another major aspect of my experience growing up was being bullied a fair amount for being abnormally pale. "Casper", "Whitey", "Powder", etc. were my nicknames. In spite of all of this I did not consider my childhood/adolescence to be unhappy and I had many joys along the way. Despite their faults my family was and is generally supportive and loving. I realize now that they were doing their best.

3. Details of your meaningful experience(s)?

I have had many, however four stick out as being the most meaningful regarding the part of my identity as being on the spectrum.

The first was my first MDMA experience at age 28. I had found a stray corgi mix that day while walking my other dog and the two dogs' faces had an uncanny resemblance despite being totally different breeds/sizes. My friend had been kind of peer-pressuring me to try Molly (MDMA) for months but I was wary of synthetics. We had plans to hang out that night and I hadn't planned on joining him on the roll but felt something strange click into place when I found this dog and just felt that it was synchronistic, which imbued me with a sense of what Joseph Campbell would label the "call to adventure."

The dog — who I assumed was being missed by someone but who I couldn't take into the humane society until the following morning because I had found him on a Sunday evening — was extremely aloof and wouldn't let me anywhere near him. I was only able to catch him in the first place because he kept wanting to play tug of war with my dog with a stick, which I used to lure him back to my backyard.

When I began peaking on Molly (MDMA), I felt a wave of soothing calm mixed with ecstatic bliss wash over me as I reclined in my lazy boy. I realized very quickly that this was in fact the first time that I could remember having absolutely no social or existential anxiety/angst. Then, all of a sudden, with my eyes still closed and rolling in the back of my head, the corgi mix stray jumped up into my lap. Something about the energy/vibe in the room had shifted and he felt safe enough to trust me finally, or so it seemed…

I felt fully whole and radically comfortable in my own skin for the first time. I'd had a few experiences with mushrooms and LSD before this that were interesting and fun but not what I would call deeply therapeutic per se. This MDMA roll was life-changing and constituted a true paradigm shift. Now I knew it was possible to feel worthy and to love myself. The next day I felt no depression or anxiety at all still and this afterglow lasted for weeks. I took the dog to the humane society assuming that his owners would be looking for him but he sat there for a week with no one searching for him so I was able to adopt him. Ghengis has been with me for 11 years now and is aging gracefully.

At age 32 I did ayahuasca just one time. The experience was incredibly intense and uncomfortable. I felt claustrophobic and disoriented the whole time. It was in an apartment and every time I opened my eyes I felt like the ceiling was directly in front of my face, so I would just shut my eyes again and repeat my mantra which I had learned from Alex Grey to employ during challenging experiences, "Observe, Allow." After everyone else had purged a bunch and they had put all the purging bowls away, I sat up to try to go pee. As soon as I did, I projectile vomited everywhere!

The shaman laughed and assured me it was ok and that it was his fault for putting the bowls away too soon. He was able to give me one to puke into soon enough for me to get some of it in there. I was able to gaze upon it and saw a dark swirling energy that felt malevolent, like a demon-eel or something. I realized that this "energy" was blocked stuff that was made of all of my petty grudges and resentments (and even revenge fantasies) towards those who had wronged me in my life. I was able to let all of that go in one purge! I was elated, to say the least. I felt physically lighter and the afterglow lasted for months. I learned the meaning of the cliche about how holding on to grudges is like carrying poison inside of you while hoping it will make your enemies sick. Such grudges only hurt me, as it turns out.

At age 35 I tried synthetic 5-MeO-DMT with the help of a guide. The guide held space masterfully and created a sacred container using ritual.

My first synthetic 5-MeO-DMT experience was basically a "white out" that I had no concrete memory of, but I was told that I lay peaceful and "buddha-like" throughout. I flew back two months later to try again and see if I could hold on to more of the experience. This time, I was more conscious of what was happening and noticed myself witnessing or observing my spirit merging with the unity of all things in a state of non-dual awareness. I was the awareness itself... I was God — and so was everything and everyone else. There was no such thing as time, but rather simply an eternal NOW. Towards the end of the experience as the ego dissolution gave way to reintegration, I became aware of the presence of the archetypal vibration of suffering. I interpreted this aspect of the experience intuitively as not to be feared, but simply to be observed with reverence and allowed to exist in a spirit of non-judgement.

I realized this was non-duality consciousness transitioning back into duality once more and that in essence that these two apparent opposites were truly just flip-sides of the same coin. They both necessitated each other. This gnosis download from the cosmos filled me with a sense of peace and acceptance of all that was, is, and will be. I was able to sit with the suffering for a while and appreciate its necessity while affirming my bodhisattva vow to work towards my sense of duty to diminish suffering in the world, and after a time (who knows how long — could have been only a few minutes in clock time but it felt much much longer) I came back to conscious awareness of my ego/body. I felt physically lighter.

The fourth most meaningful trip was my first time doing a ketamine IV infusion. All the myriad details are a bit hazy due to the dissociative's adverse effects on memory — it seemed to last for ages while I was in the k-hole and there were many many layers of experience — but what stuck with me was that I had a "reactivation" of my recent 5-MeO-DMT experience (also sometimes called a "re-galactivation"). I felt truly held by the divine archetypal feminine aspect of the universe that I identified as Nuit. This was at the beginning of the trip.

After a few minutes of laughing and crying and saying "thank you, thank you!" I "sunk down" into a deeper layer of the k-hole. I can only describe this feeling as reaching some sort of sunken place or null point. I felt like I was at the nexus of the universe and that there was no coming back. I felt like I had "locked-in syndrome" and that my body was a lifeless husk. It was at this time that I had the thought that I had died and I was absolutely convinced of this fact. In my panic, I shifted into a vision where I was a heroin addict who had overdosed. I was me, but also not me. Like a bad nightmare. I somehow understood that I had truly messed up for the last time and that the ambulance was on its way to pick up my corpse and that my parents were going to be so deeply affected and disappointed in me for what they would view as throwing my life away.

Then, there was another shift into another layer. I accepted my fate and made peace with it, having remembered from a PhD anecdote that this was the wise thing to do in such a scenario. As soon as I stopped panicking and accepted my fate I was reborn like a glorious phoenix and realized that this was just all an alchemical transmutation of my spirit. It had been necessary in order for me to fully integrate my 5-MeO-DMT experiences in a more conscious and intentional way, so that I could truly feel initiated like the legends of those who underwent the Eleusinian Mysteries. I have felt to my core since that day that I do not fear death and that it is to be embraced and even looked forward to when it is my time to transition to the next adventure. I realized it was all always going to be OK and that I was here to help others heal now that I had found my healing for my core-wounding.

4. Reaction / integration related to these meaningful psychedelic experience(s)?

I guess I kinda already covered this in my long-winded replies above lol

5. Feelings toward the psychedelic experience(s) over time?

I feel less need to have these experiences as frequently these days and feel like I have, in a sense, gotten "the message" so it's ok to hang up the receiver! That said, just for routine ego maintenance I still like to do some sort of trip every 6 months or so. I do so now in a very sacred and reverent way every time with lots of intention and attention to integration.

6. Notable challenges/difficulties of your experiences?

Covered this haha

7. Perceived or lasting benefits of your psychedelic experiences?

I know in my heart that I am worthy of love now. I know that I am here to serve and to love all of life. I will never let my inner critic hold sway and influence me to believe that I am not enough. I truly believe that I have a sacred duty to help alleviate suffering.

8. In one sentence, how would you summarize what happened & why it is important?

Para el bien de todos. [For the good of all.]

9. What's next for you in this exploration?

I have a growing confidence that I can become a veritable "neo-shaman" through using my recently-completed counseling graduate degree to help others by holding space for their journeys and/or with integration work. I have the confidence to embark on the PhD in transpersonal psychology program that I will be starting this Spring at my school. I will eventually become a psychedelic-assisted psychotherapist and/or researcher.

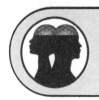

Catalina's Words

Content Warning: Discussion of Suicidal Ideation

1. Bio (name, age, home country, diagnosis if applicable)

Catalina. Age 32, Ecuador, Asperger's Syndrome.

2. How did you feel / behave in the years before your psychedelic experiences (growing up, socially, etc)

Growing up was really difficult. I never quite understood why I was so different, and at first I thought I was damaged. It was so difficult for me to make friends or understand how to behave as a child, and also as a teenager. I used to experiment with people in order to discover different outcomes and use that information in future interactions — although now that I think about it, that was not ethical at all, but I was a child and I didn't know better.

I was always really smart and one of the best students at school. I participated in advanced programs and got good grades but socially I never understood a thing. I remember my mom telling me she thought I was dumb because I did not understand a lot of social situations, and the communication barrier I experienced was so literal. I had to learn all the expressions by memory because I live in a country that uses so many figures of speech that do not make any sense.

I couldn't control my emotions, or even identify them, I believe I grew up with anxiety and sadness until I was 23, which was near to the age in which I tried psychedelics for the first time. I have always been hypersensitive. I couldn't eat food if the texture was irregular, or if any of the food components got mixed up. I could not tolerate rugged textures. I could not tolerate loud noises such as the lawn mower or the blender. I remember that It was always easy for me to socialize with animals, and it still is.

At family reunions I used to be by myself, or with the animals. I cried most of my adolescence because I felt really sad, I even had suicidal thoughts and tried to commit suicide twice. I had very specific interests my whole life including ancient civilizations, astronomy, megalithic constructions, and consciousness, all from a very young age. My dream was to invent a machine that could decode human consciousness, and I guess I found that sacred technology in entheogens.

I used to be an atheist and very narrow minded. I always thought that the only things that were true were the things you could prove with the scientific method and I would always correct people on how they spoke, or how they wrote, or how correct I felt the content of what they were saying might have been. I used to be very arrogant and got easily offended by pretty much anything. I had a very hard time identifying which emotions belonged to me and what belonged to others, and I would easily project my own problems onto others, and there was no way that anybody was going to convince me that I was not right. Yes. I thought I was the smartest person in the room and I really liked making sure everybody knew that. This is not something I do not feel pride toward.

In time, I accepted my own process of growing up and I am very glad that I got an opportunity to better myself and get more in touch with the divinity within me that lets me see the divinity within everyone else. Before psychedelics, my cognitive functions were a mess, my reward system was out of balance, and I could not make decisions based on a long term outcome because I would always choose immediate pleasure. I had difficulty recognizing potentially dangerous situations. I thought I could do it all by myself. I did a lot of reckless things growing up that put my life in danger.

3. Details of your meaningful experience(s)?

I can't recall which psychedelic I tried first, but over the course of a certain period of time I tried San Pedro or Wachuma (Echinopsis pachanoi), Peyote (Lophophora williamsii), LSD, & mushrooms. I started to have the ability to perceive myself as if I was an outside observer which let me have great insight on all of my processes.

At around the same time I started to learn Sacred Geometry, magic, numerology, and all of the sudden everything started changing. It was a gradual process then, and it still is now. Over time I started seeing synchronicities every single day, with the numbers and the events, and the words, as if everything was perfectly designed by some great architect.

I went to med school and became a doctor — although I still have trouble with western medicine because it is so limited — and that has had a deep impact on me. I began learning astrology and having the capability to identify archetypes in myself. I know that all of the knowledge came with the use of entheogens, because before I rejected all of that information because the scientific method could never prove it.

I have experienced more than 100 psychedelic sessions. I am fortunate to live in a country where this is sacred patrimony. I have also tried many synthetic compounds that can be found here too.

Every single session has been meaningful for me. It is like going to therapy for a month, in a single session. I have cried, laughed, danced, thrown up, felt desperate, felt part of the universe. I have visited different realities, I have seen beings that have told me I am on the right path. I guide myself with synchronicities now, I communicate with numbers that show me the way.

Everything changed for me, I began understanding the patterns of behavior that had shaped my life, my own behavior. I could see those patterns reflected on my family and how that had affected me. It's as if I gained a superpower to see inside of myself. In such a graphic way, I saw the cartography of my own psyche. I spent a lot of time reading about psychology and non-ordinary states of consciousness in order to decipher my own self and be able to help myself because no psychologist or psychiatrist ever could do so. Entheogens shattered my defense mechanisms, although no one knew because I always kept this to myself. I tried telling my mom but she always thought I was making excuses to drug myself. I gradually saw changes. I then went on to study Ancestral Sciences, Reiki, and I am now on the Transpersonal Training program in South America. All of these happened because of my exposure to psychedelics and non-ordinary states of consciousness.

I still am healing because it is such a long journey. I want to become a psychiatrist to be able to help people who have had similar diagnoses as mine. I love working with the Kyron archetype of the wounded Healer. The best way to help myself is through helping others and the only way to be able to help others is to heal myself first.

4. Reactions / Integration related to these meaningful psychedelic experience(s)?

My life changed completely, I am in love with non-ordinary states of consciousness and their therapeutic potential and will dedicate my life to studying, practicing, and serving others with these tools.

5. Feelings toward the psychedelic experience(s) over time?

I will compare non-ordinary states of consciousness with driving a spaceship. It is as if I learned to drive and it is easy to navigate now. No matter the substance, I am always very present, very focused, and very aware of the details inside of me and around me.

6. Notable challenges/difficulties of your experiences?

I have become too sensitive to LSD and MDMA, I feel my body intoxicated sometimes, it is as if the acid is too strong for my body. I prefer natural entheogens now.

7. Perceived or lasting benefits of your psychedelic experiences?

- Introspection
- Ability to navigate with my own emotions in an adequate way
- Ability to see myself as an outside observer
- Reward system is finally in equilibrium
- Emotional stability
- Ability to make decisions based on a long-term benefits
- Sense of well-being & bliss
- Feeling connected to everyone & everything
- A LOT of empathy
- Extreme ability to see patterns
- Extreme ability to recognize synchronicities with numbers & symbols

8. In one sentence, how would you summarize what happened & why it is important?

I was able to access the cartography of my own psyche and began working on my own biographical, perinatal and transpersonal issues. It is important to understand the way we were constructed and what archetypes and behavioral patterns are shaping our experience in order to be able to modify them.

9. What's next for you in this exploration?

I have not tried Bufo Alvarius yet. I am waiting to vibrate in that frequency so that the universe presents an opportunity for me to receive this medicine. I am trying to heal because I got sick 2 years ago, and I now have Myofascial Syndrome which is the most horrible thing that has happened to me. I want to find out if fascia can be modified and regenerated with the use of DMT.

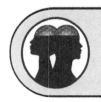 # Suzanne's Words

1. Bio (age, home country, diagnosis if applicable)

Suzanne. Age 32, USA, Autism Spectrum Disorder and ADHD

2. How did you feel / behave in the years before your psychedelic experiences (growing up, socially, etc)

I had my first psychedelic experience when I was 22 years old but before that, growing up, I would rarely make eye contact with other people, especially if I didn't know them super well. I was considered sweet, shy, quirky, creative, and super sensitive (emotionally & physically). My parents and their culture have a huge stigma against autism, so I wasn't diagnosed until this current year, 2020. Teachers would tell my parents that I wouldn't really make eye contact. I never participated in class so I was put into a gifted program at 8 years old because of my advanced reading skills at the time, but I was kicked out soon after. I fell behind in math at a young age and don't think I've ever fully recovered. Also, I was very rigid about right and wrong and had a strong sense of environmental and social justice.

As a child, I had a really hard time making and keeping friends. My parents put me in a lot of school activities like sports and Girl Scouts, which helped me socialize. However, around 7 or 8 years old I started experiencing existential crises regularly and would often come home heartbroken because I didn't understand why I was always one of the last picked for groups in class or why most of the other kids didn't seem to want to be friends with me. The 8-year-old me believed this was due to the way I looked or that something was wrong with me. I started to overthink social interactions even more which did not help me socially and gave me anxiety. Additionally, I was always getting injured and losing things. I wound up on crutches several times between the age of 10 and 15, once for tripping up the stairs and spraining my ankles.

As a teenager, I developed depression, anxiety, and an eating disorder. The friends I had were always other girls my age with dominant personalities that I could piggyback off socially as I hid behind their extroversion and loudness. I learned at a very early age — like 8 years old or younger — to mask and hide my autistic traits as well as any behavior that could be received by other people as "weird" because I noticed that I was starting to be left out amongst my peers in school.

I'd usually be friends with other girls who had more extroverted personalities and liked to take up space and would mimic my peers to figure out how to behave in social situations. Masking served me in the sense that it protected me from being bullied socially, which still happened once in a while. But I'm definitely more unhappy and feel inauthentic if I'm masking all of the time.

It wasn't until I started experimenting with entheogens and empathogens that I truly became aware that the emotions and feelings in my head weren't translating in my facial expressions or tone of voice. It had been pointed out to me here and there, but I never really believed it because I wasn't experiencing myself that way. Also, it wasn't until I experienced psychedelics that I felt like I could connect with all of my brain and other people more fully.

3. Details of your meaningful experience(s)?

At this point in life I've had a lot of meaningful experiences that have taught me something new about myself and others. The first time I did MDMA, I felt seen and understood by my neurotypical friends in a way that I hadn't experienced previously and vice versa. Just the other day, I recounted the experience with my friend — who shared this entheogenic experience with me for my first time — and how it helped us individually and our friendship. I learned more about actively listening to other people and that at the end of the day, neurodivergent and neurotypical people both want to connect, to be understood, and to love and be loved. It can be very difficult for me to make new friendships and maintain them, but I feel like MDMA has assisted me in more clearly communicating my experience emotionally to my friend. Like many autistic people, I struggle with being socially naive and figuring out other people's intentions and motivations

Another meaningful experience that taught me a lot and provided a lot of healing was with ayahuasca when I was about 24 years old. I had been in recovery from an eating disorder for over a decade when I the drank ayahuasca, and part of my experience involved me feeling the need to vomit and feeling so much shame around it, because so much shame was tied into purging from my eating disorder and having bulimic tendencies. So while I felt seasick I crawled to the bathroom, barely shut the door, and puked out what looked like galaxies in the universe. All of a sudden the thing I felt so ashamed about was beautiful, and I understood that it was an opportunity to heal. I got up, looked in the mirror, and saw a wild woman, who looked almost feral with markings on her face. Her eyes looked so alive and she was vital. She looked like me, but stronger. I went back to lie down in my spot near the shaman and held my abdomen like a baby. I heard a voice whispering, "Heal," and I felt more at peace with myself than I ever had before. I felt all of my parents' love and all of the love the universe has for me and all beings.

4. Reaction / integration related to these meaningful psychedelic experience(s)?

Psychedelics and spirit medicine are useful catalysts for people — whether they're autistic or not — who are seeking to explore their mind, emotions, and connection. They're amazing teachers because they work in conjunction with the way your mind works and the substances themselves expand your perception — at least that's how it feels to me. It is in this place of expanded perception that I can more easily connect and communicate with others. This expanded state of perception is also where I experience more compassion for myself and others. I feel like psychedelics have taught me so much about myself and have helped me to work through personal struggles and helped me to connect the dots in my life so I can keep learning how to grow as a person.

5. Feelings toward the psychedelic experience(s) over time?

I was terrified of psychedelics and plant spirit medicine for a very long time. I was terrified of losing any sort of control of my mind or developing brain damage. I grew up with the D.A.R.E. (Drug Abuse Resistance Education) Program in school which told me that all drugs are bad and cannabis is a gateway drug to the bad drugs.

It's very funny to me now that I've experienced a very different reality than what I was taught during D.A.R.E. Some substances, like psilocybin mushrooms and MDMA, are actually beneficial if taken intentionally and safely.

I was very naive about psychedelics when I began exploring with them, so I tried DMT as one of my first and nothing really seemed scary after that. This is not to say that I had a negative experience — in fact, quite the contrary.

The DMT experience was one of the most vivid and beautiful experiences I've ever had.

6. Notable challenges/difficulties of your experiences?

The setting matters a lot. I tried to take LSD at a party once and ended up with anxiety for most of it and wanted to be alone. The energy and environment around me influences how my experiences with psychedelics flow and affect me, so intention and setting are important.

7. Perceived or lasting benefits of your psychedelic experiences?

I'm kinder towards myself. Although I'm still improving and still experience struggles, I feel like I'm better at communicating my feelings now.

8. In one sentence, how would you summarize what happened & why it is important?

My perception expanded, I connected with so many layers of my humanity, I healed years of trauma, and the quality of my life improved.

9. What's next for you in this exploration?

Being gentle with myself while also challenging myself. I still plan on using various plant medicines as part of my self-care and personal growth practice.

Time will tell what they'll teach me next.

THE CONVERSATION CONTINUES...

by Aaron Paul Orsini

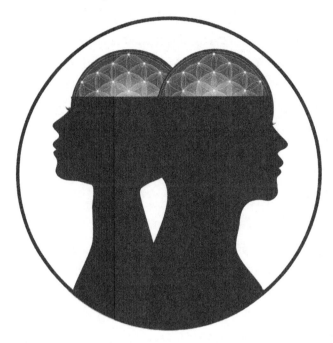

Psychedelic molecules are like fire. Yes. And the contributors of this publication have offered up their words to explain the significance of their encounters with that fire; to remind readers and the rest of the world that the fire can heal; the fire can warm; and yes, the fire can potentially harm. But the potential harms and risks and dangers of this fire are only ever as real as our own naivety, and our own lack of respect and knowledge related to the potentially intense power of the psychedelic flame.

And so, here we are, the humbled recipients of that flame — a flame that has impacted us all in such a wide variety of ways.

For some, this flame has kept us warm during the darkest and coldest of nights. For others, this flame has illuminated this same darkness to show us the light and beauty and potential of this life, this planet, this human family, and beyond. And if that all sounds a bit too cosmic to consider, I remind us all that some of us have also used the flame to help us simply function better during times in which we needed a little bit of light in order to perceive ourselves or others more clearly.

Regardless of the size of the fire we choose to ignite, or the choice of kindling, or the intentions of those who have wielded the psychedelic flame in whatever ways that have served them best, I feel comfortably confident in stating that the contributors of this book are all united and bound together by the same essential truth, and that is this: we have each perceived some benefit in having encountered this flame. This is not to say that all of the potential risks involved in wielding this flame do not exist. They do. And this is also why it's critical to host discussions of this sort — so that we can continue to combine insights and perpetually refine approaches to reduce any and all risks over time.

In the end, our personally relevant outcomes may or may not translate to others. Nevertheless, our personal truths and experiences remain valid — always.

There is so much more to learn, and so many more stories to be shared. And it is my sincere hope that the publishing of this book has helped to provide a glimpse of why the continuous fostering of this discussion might be of tremendous importance to many, many people.

This is complicated. All of this is complicated. I know. But if we decide to continue to meaningfully participate in this dialogue — and build upon the preliminary foundations of understanding that have been put forth through the publishing of this book — then we will likewise grant ourselves permission to discover what's possible when we set aside the stigmas and make space for sincere and peaceable listening.

And so on behalf of all those who have contributed to this publication, I extend one last expression of gratitude, to you, the reader, for your attention, your time, and your interest in the words that have been offered here in this book.

If you have any thoughts or insights you would like to contribute to this collaborative discussion, we welcome you to do so anytime via the forums, meetings, and surveys hosted at AutisticPsychedelic.com.

We'd appreciate hearing from you. And maybe others would, too.

May all beings be peaceful.

May all beings be safe.

With Love & Gratitude,

Aaron Paul Orsini

Co-Organizer @

Autistic Psychedelic Community

CONTINUED READING (NEURODIVERGENCE)

The Power of Neurodiversity:
Unleashing The Advantages of
Your Differently Wired Brain
Thomas Armstrong, PhD

Asperger's From the Inside Out:
A Supportive and Practical Guide for
Anyone with Asperger's Syndrome
Michael John Carley

The Spectrum Girl's Survival Guide:
How to Grow Up Awesome & Autistic
Siena Castellon

A Field Guide to Earthlings:
An Autistic/Asperger View of Neurotypical Behavior
Ian Ford

I Think I Might Be Autistic:
A Guide To Autism Spectrum Disorder
Diagnosis & Self-Discovery for Adults
Cynthia Kim

Plankton Dreams:
What I Learned in Special Ed
Tito Rajarshi Mukhopadhyay

Divergent Mind:
Thriving in a World That Wasn't Designed For You
Jenara Nerenberg

CONTINUED READING (NEURODIVERGENCE)

Scholars With Autism Achieving Dreams
Lars Perner, PhD

Care Work: Dreaming Disability Justice
Leah Lakshmi Piepzna-Samarasinha

Laziness Does Not Exist
Devon Price, PhD

Switched On:
A Memoir of Brain Change
& Emotional Awakening
John Elder Robinson

Neurotribes:
The Legacy of Autism & The Future of Neurodiversity
Steve Silberman

Spectrums:
Autistic Transgender People in Their Own Words
Maxfield Sparrow

Born On A Blue Day:
Inside The Extraordinary Mind
Of An Autistic Savant
Daniel Tammet

Disability Visibility:
First-Person Stories from the Twenty-First Century
Alice Wong

CONTINUED READING (PSYCHEDELICS)

Consciousness Medicine:
Indigenous Wisdom, Entheogens &
Expanded States of Consciousness for Healing & Growth
Francoise Bourzat

Frontiers of Psychedelic Consciousness:
Conversations with Albert Hofmann, Stanislav Grof,
Rick Strassman, Jeremy Narby, Simon Posford & Others
David Brown

The Psychedelic Explorer's Guide
James Fadiman, PhD

Good Chemistry:
The Science of Connection, From Soul to Psychedelics
Julie Holland, MD

Handbook of Medical Hallucinogens
Charles S. Grob, MD, Jim Grigsby, PhD

LSD Psychotherapy
Stanislav Grof MD, PhD, Albert Hoffman, PhD

LSD My Problem Child:
Reflections on Sacred Drugs, Mysticism & Science
Albert Hoffman, PhD

Your Psilocybin Mushroom Companion:
An Informative, Easy-to-Use Guide to Understanding Magic Mushrooms
— From Tips & Trips to Microdosing & Psychedelic Therapy
Michelle Janikian

CONTINUED READING (PSYCHEDELICS)

Neuropsychedelia:
The Revival of Hallucinogen Research
Since The Decade of The Brain
Nicolas Langlitz

Changing Our Minds:
Psychedelic Sacraments & The New Psychotherapy
Don Lattin

Psychedelic Medicine:
The Healing Powers of LSD, MDMA, Psilocybin & Ayahuasca
Richard Louise Miller, MA, PhD

Drugs Without The Hot Air:
Making Sense of Legal & Illegal Drugs
David Nutt, PhD

Autism On Acid:
How LSD Helped Me Understand, Navigate,
Alter & Appreciate My Autistic Perceptions
Aaron Paul Orsini

The Science of Microdosing Psychedelics
Torsten Passie, MD, PhD

How to Change Your Mind:
What The New Science of Psychedelics Teaches Us About Consciousness,
Dying, Addiction, Depression & Transcendence
Michael Pollan

PiHKAL: A Chemical Love Story & TiHKAL: The Continuation
Alexander Shulgrin, PhD

The Wild Kindness: A Psilocybin Odyssey
Bett Williams

INDEX

To Join This Collaboration, Please Visit

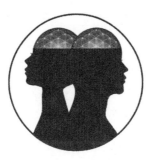

AUTISTICPSYCHEDELIC.COM

Or Discuss This Book Using Hashtag
#AutisticPsychedelic
On Social Media...

Twitter.com/AutisticPsyched

Reddit.com/r/AutisticPsychedelic

Instagram.com/AutisticPsychedelic

TikTok.com/@AutisticPsychedelic

...And If You Found This Book To Be Insightful In Any Way,
Please Consider Donating 30 Seconds of Your Time
To Write Us A Review :)

AutisticPsychedelic.com/review

Printed in Great Britain
by Amazon

20377790R00106